Coronary Heart Disease Prevention

Coronary Heart Disease Prevention

Plans for Action

A report based on an interdisciplinary workshop conference held at Canterbury on 28–30 September 1983

PITMAN

First Published 1984

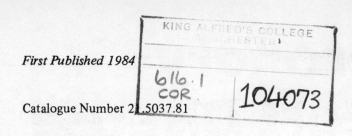

Catalogue Number 21.5037.81

Pitman Publishing Ltd
128 Long Acre
London WC2E 9AN

Associated Companies
Pitman Publishing Pty Ltd, Melbourne
Pitman Publishing New Zealand Ltd, Wellington

British Library Cataloguing in Publication Data

Coronary heart disease prevention.
    1. Coronary heart disease—Prevention
    616.1'2305   RC685.C6

ISBN 0-272-79789-8

Printed and bound in Great Britain by
Biddles Ltd, Guildford and King's Lynn

ACKNOWLEDGMENTS

The copyright to the 'Canterbury' Report has been assigned to the Health Education Council. Authorship of the report lies with the Steering Committee who are listed below, and therefore does not necessarily represent the views of the Sponsors, Co-sponsors or participants.

Geoffrey Rose (Chairman)
Keith Ball
John Catford
Philip James
Deryck Lambert
Alan Maryon-Davis
Michael Oliver
David Player
Christopher Robbins
Alwyn Smith

LIST OF SPONSORS AND CO-SPONSORS

The Canterbury conference was sponsored by:

- The Health Education Council (who also funded the conference)
- The Department of Health and Social Security (in association with the health departments of Scotland, Northern Ireland and Wales)
- The British Cardiac Society
- The Coronary Prevention Group (who also gave administrative and secretarial support)

A wide range of other professional bodies also agreed to be co-sponsors:

- Action on Smoking and Health
- British Dietetic Association
- British Heart Foundation
- British Medical Association
- Chest, Heart and Stroke Association
- Faculty of Community Medicine
- Faculty of Occupational Medicine
- Health Visitors' Association
- Royal College of General Practitioners
- Royal College of Nursing
- Royal College of Physicians (Edinburgh)
- Royal College of Physicians (London)
- Royal College of Physicians and Surgeons (Glasgow)
- Scottish Health Education Group
- Society of Health Education Officers
- Sports Council
- Trades Union Congress

LIST OF CONTRIBUTORS AND MEMBERS OF CONFERENCE COMMITTEES

Dr Sheila Adam
Brent Health Authority

Dr Richard Alderslade
Department of Health and Social Security

Dr John Ashton
Department of Community Health, Liverpool University

Ms Lorna Bailey
Centre for Continuing Education, Open University

Dr Keith Ball
Department of Community Medicine, Central Middlesex Hospital, London. *Member of Steering Committee*

Mr Alan Beattie
Institute of Education, University of London. *Convenor and Member of Programme Committee*

Dr Nick Bradley
General Practitioner, Exeter

Professor D Britton
Wye College

Mr Martin Buxton
Health Economics Research, Brunel University

Mr Geoffrey Cannon
"Sunday Times"

Dr John Catford
Wessex Regional Health Authority. *Member of Steering Committee, Convenor and Member of Programme Committee*

Professor David Chambers
London Business School, University of London

Mr R Charmen
Oxford Regional Health Authority

Mr David Cohen
Health Economics Research, Aberdeen University

Ms Issy Cole-Hamilton
West Lambeth Health Authority

Mr Mike Daube
Department of Community Medicine, Usher Institute, Edinburgh University

Mr Stuart Dickens
South Birmingham Health Authority

Mrs Alison Dobson
Brent Health Authority

Dr Peter Draper
Unit for the study of Health policy, Guy's Hospital Medical School

Dr Jack Edelman
Lord Rank Research Centre

Ms Annabel Ferriman
"The Observer". *Convenor and Member of Programme Committee*

Dr Alex Gatherer
Oxfordshire Health Authority

Dr Donald Gau
General Practitioner, Beaconsfield.
Convenor and Member of Programme Committee

Ms Shirley Goodwin
Health Visitors' Association

Dr Andrew Haines
General Practitioner, Harlesden

Ms Carol Haslam
Channel 4 Television

Dr Julian Tudor Hart
General Practitioner, Glyncorrwg

Professor Alan Henderson
National School of Medicine, University of Wales

Mr Ivor Hunt
J Sainsbury Marketing Services

Dr Sandra Hunt
Nutritionist, London

Dr Philip James
Rowett Research Institute, Aberdeen. *Member of Steering Committee,*
Chairman of Programme Committee and Workshop

Miss Sue Jenkins
Community Health Council, Leeds

Mr Lewis Jollans
Centre for Agricultural Strategy, Reading University

Ms Lesley Jones
Bradford and Airedale Health Authority Education Unit

Professor R Klein
University of Bath

Dr Deryck Lambert
Department of Health and Social Security.
Member of Steering Committee

Dr John Lawson
Royal College of General Practitioners.
Workshop Chairman

Dr J Mann
Department of Community Medicine, Oxford

Mr Robin McCron
Centre for Mass Communication Research,
Leicester University

Dr Alan Maryon-Davis
Health Education Council.
Member of Steering Committee

Professor Jerry Morris
London School of Hygiene and Tropical Medicine.
Convenor and Member of Programme Committee

Dr Sue Mowatt
Tower Hamlets Health Authority

Professor Risteard Mulcahy
St Vincent's Hospital, Dublin

Dr Frank Murphy
West Essex Health Authority

Mr Don Nutbeam
Wessex Regional Health Authority

Dr Michael O'Donnell
Journalist. *Workshop Chairman*

Professor Michael Oliver
Cardiovascular Research, Edinburgh University.
Member of Steering Committee

Ms Susan Owens
"Woman's Own"

Mr Richard Parish
Stockport Health Authority

Dr D Parken
Area Medical Officers' Association

Dr Pereira Gray
General Practitioner, Exeter

Dr Zbynek Pisa
World Health Organization

Dr David Player
Health Education Council.
Member of Steering Committee

Professor Kalevi Pyörälä
Kuopio University, Finland

Professor Frank Raymond
Formerly Ministry of Agriculture

Mr Don Reid
Health Education Council

Mr Christopher Robbins
Coronary Prevention Group, London.
Member of Steering Committee, Conference Secretary

Dr John Rook
Agricultural Research Council.
Workshop Chairman

Professor Geoffrey Rose
London School of Hygiene and Tropical Medicine.
Conference Chairman, Chairman of Steering Committee

Mr Howard Seymour
Manchester Health Education Department

Dr Roger Skinner
Department of Health and Social Security

Professor Alwyn Smith
University Hospital of South Manchester.
Member of Steering Committee

Professor Colin Spedding
Department of Agriculture and Horticulture, Reading University.
Convenor and Member of Programme Committee

Dr K Taylor
Formerly Health Education Council

Ms Jane Thomas
Queen Elizabeth College, University of London

Ms June Thompson
Health Visitors' Association

Mr Howard Wagstaff
Department of Agricultural Economics, Edinburgh University

Miss Caroline Walker
City and Hackney Health Authority

Mr Geoff Watts
BBC

Mr Nick Wells
Office of Health Economics, London

Mr Kingsley Williams
Former Chairman, Wessex Regional Health Authority.
Workshop Chairman

SUMMARY

On 28–30 September 1983 a workshop conference was held at the University of Kent, Canterbury to consider practical ways in which the World Health Organization's recommendations on the prevention of coronary heart disease could be rapidly implemented in the United Kingdom. Coronary heart disease today places an enormous burden on the nation in both human and economic terms. There appears to be considerable scope for reducing the incidence of the disease if the problems of smoking, an unhealthy diet and too little exercise can be tackled. The UK now has some of the highest rates of premature death from coronary heart disease in the world and has not experienced a decline in deaths like that of many of the developed countries. Urgent action is required.

Eighty people contributed to the Canterbury Conference, either through preparing pre-conference working documents or attending workshops. They represented a wide range of disciplines and had considerable expertise in the fields of national policy, food and agriculture, National Health Service, primary health care, health education, or the mass media. The conference was sponsored by the Health Education Council, Department of Health and Social Security (in association with other UK Health Departments), the British Cardiac Society and the Coronary Prevention Group. Many other professional bodies also lent their support.

This report has been prepared by the Steering Committee and is based on the discussions of the conference. It brings together for the first time the wide range of issues involved and makes proposals for practical steps through which progress could be made in the short to medium term. The report seeks to stimulate discussion at every level about ways to achieve energetic and comprehensive action to reduce the huge load that coronary heart disease places on the British people.

The following summarise the practically-orientated recommendations made in the report which relate to both a population approach and the identification of high risk groups. They are not necessarily in order of priority.

1. A National strategy for the prevention of coronary heart disease should now be established. This should state the objectives and targets that are sought by the various organisations and interest groups that influence directly or indirectly the major risk factors. In addition to policy statements, specific programmes will need

xii

to be developed for smoking control, healthy nutrition, and exercise promotion. Following careful economic assessment, sufficient resources should be made available. In the context of the Department of Health and the National Health Service the prevention of coronary heart disease should become a major priority. The Department of Education and Science should also give this increased importance, especially in schools.

2. Within central government as a whole the health consequences of economic and other developments should be fully considered so that the promotion of health becomes a major national priority. To this end the Department of Health should establish a 'watchdog' Standing Committee and a seat should be created on the National Economic Development Council for a health representative.

3. The prevention and control of smoking should receive more energetic support from central government along the lines recommended by the Royal College of Physicians, i.e. in the fields of taxation, availability and sales promotion. There should be no attempt to promote the consumption of so-called 'safer cigarettes'.

4. Coronary heart disease prevention should be promoted in a co-ordinated and complementary way by existing national organisations, such as the Royal Colleges, the British Cardiac Society, the British Heart Foundation, the Coronary Prevention Group, the Health Education Council and the Departments of Health. A working party should be formed as a matter of urgency to discuss how progress can be made.

5. Professional bodies, universities and training colleges have a major responsibility to ensure that both health and education professionals are appropriately trained in prevention. Urgent attention should be given to pre- and post-qualification teaching and in-service training. The Sports Council, health charities, voluntary organisations, the Confederation of British Industry, and the trades union movement, should also lend their active support to prevention on a wide number of fronts.

6. The promotion of healthy nutrition should receive a higher priority within the Ministry of Agriculture, Fisheries and Food. Those elements of the Common Agricultural Policy counter to healthy food policy should be opposed. Ministers should also use their opportunities to ensure that the European Economic Community

addresses itself more to health and specifically the prevention of coronary heart disease.

7. UK government policy should ensure that the food and agricultural industries are encouraged towards production of healthy foods. Codes of practice relating to fat, sugar and salt content of manufactured food, and sales promotion practices should be evolved in ways which are sensitive to economic realities. There should be far greater public participation in policy decisions about increasing the availability of healthy foods. There also needs to be clear and simple food labelling.

8. The Health Education Council and Scottish Health Education Group have already made important contributions to the development of preventive programmes. More work is required in the fields of information, co-ordination and support, particularly training, development of curricula and materials, and mass media initiatives. The Council should become more regionally orientated to ensure joint planning with other organisations along the lines of its Welsh Heart Programme. To undertake these additional activities the Departments of Health should provide more resources and staff. An increase of at least £8 million per annum is recommended for these organisations to undertake heart disease prevention programmes in the United Kingdom.

9. Regional and District Health Authorities should recognise their crucial and unique role in the prevention of coronary heart disease and should be held accountable for ensuring that progress is made. Developments should be one of the highest priorities for available health service expenditure. To stimulate activity at a time of financial constraint 'pump-priming' grants should be provided for health authorities by the Departments of Health. An injection of £12 million per annum (less than 0.1 per cent of total health service spending) is recommended to ensure action within health authorities in the United Kingdom.

10. Regional and District Health Authorities should incorporate prevention of coronary heart disease into core planning and delivery of health services. Plans should state overall policies and priorities, the programmes that will be mounted to achieve specified objectives and targets, and the resources, infrastructure and the form of monitoring that will be used. There should be better communication between bodies at all levels to ensure joint planning and execution of programmes.

11. Input at local community level, both lay and professional, should be an essential part of planning and implementing programmes for the prevention of coronary heart disease. Neighbourhood groups for health promotion need to be encouraged and supported. At District level there should be an interdisciplinary Heart Disease Prevention Team providing steering and co-ordination. The Team should have a budget so that new schemes and projects within the community can be initiated.

12. All members of the Primary Health Care Team should accept their important responsibility in the prevention of coronary heart disease. This will include the prevention and control of smoking, obesity and hypertension, and the promotion of exercise and healthy nutrition. An anticipatory as well as reactive approach is required. The appointment of a liaison person to stimulate, support and co-ordinate activities is essential.

13. Preventive activities of the Primary Health Care Team should be encouraged and supported by the development of patient participation groups, better systems of practice organisation, greater involvement in research, and increased health visitor and nurse input. There need to be better team skills, more flexibility in professional roles and improved links with health education officers, dietitians and other groups. Provision of training at every stage and level is essential together with supportive literature and manuals etc.

14. In addition to general public education and encouraging community action, Primary Health Care Teams should direct activities towards identifying high risk individuals, where prevention can be particularly effective. This requires the development of better information systems within primary care which should be the responsibility of an identified Team member. Additional resources may be necessary from the District. There should also be regularly published practice reports which should act as both a stimulus for the Team and the local community, and as an important source for the compilation of a District health profile.

15. Health education approaches should include the provision of health risk advice to individuals, raising public awareness about health issues, encouraging personal self-esteem and self-empowerment, and developing community action. The wide range of opportunities and settings for health education at local level should be used to

the full − in schools, adult and community education centres, the workplace, and primary health care. Support at District, Regional and National level should be available, particularly in the provision of resources, support materials and training, and in the development and co-ordination of mass media initiatives.

16. At District level the development of health education policies, programmes and training courses, as well as careful co-ordination of activities is required. A multi-disciplinary steering group for health education should be established as a sub-group of the District Heart Disease Prevention Team. A health education officer should be appointed in each District to work in the field of community action development. District Health Education Units are fundamental for success, and the majority of Units in the UK need to be considerably strengthened.

17. Local Education Authorities should give their active support to the development of health education in schools, and within adult and community education. Co-ordinators need to be identified, who should be concerned not only with formal educational activities but also with the 'hidden' curriculum which can be counterproductive (e.g. staff smoking, unhealthy school meals, etc). The Health Education Council should continue to develop appropriate curricula, teaching packs and training courses for teachers.

18. The Media should accept their important responsibility for promoting and protecting the nation's health. They should avoid encouraging confrontation if it leads to confusion. Each media organisation should identify a health correspondent. The BBC and IBA should produce internal documents on their roles in safeguarding the nation's health. To capture media interest there should be a 'Year of the Heart', regular press conferences, briefing documents and newsletters and sponsored health events. The Coronary Prevention Group should play an active part here.

19. To aid better communication between media and health professionals, the Health Education Council should extend its role in providing names of appropriate individuals and agencies who can give advice. The Council should also sponsor National Press awards for 'Best Health Coverage'. In general the media should be used more purposefully, and this will require better training and equipping of health professionals. National Health Service press and public relations departments should substantially develop

their activities in health promotion. Co-ordination of mass media and community based programmes is vital.

20. There should be much greater investment in research relating to the means and effectiveness of preventing coronary heart disease. Improved monitoring of preventive programmes within the agricultural and food industries and the National Health Service, as well as in local communities is essential. Government should ensure that sufficient resources have been made available to assess the speed of progress, so that alternative strategies can be implemented where necessary.

CONTENTS

Acknowledgments   *iii*

List of Sponsors and Co-sponsors   *v*

List of Contributors and Members of Conference Committees   *vii*

Summary   *xi*

1. Introduction   1

    The Need for Action   1
    The Canterbury Conference and Report   3

2. Action at National Level   5

    European Economic Community   5
    UK Government   6
    Development of a National Strategy   6
    National Organisations   7
    Controlling the Smoking Epidemic   9
    Recommendations   9

3. Action Within the Food and Agricultural Industries   12

    Dietary Goals for Agriculture   12
    Ministry of Agriculture, Fisheries and Food   14
    Consumer Attitudes and Needs   16
    Research and Development   17
    Recommendations   17

4. Action Through the National Health Service   20

    Role of the National Health Service   20
    Development of Planning and Monitoring   21
    Importance of Local Input   21
    Funding Sources and Mechanisms   22
    Recommendations   23

5. Action Within Primary Health Care   30

    Role of the Primary Health Care Team   30
    Motivating the Primary Health Care Team   31
    Recommendations   33

6. Action Through Health Education   40

    Choice of Health Education Approaches   40
    Organisational Aspects   42
    Role of Key Agencies   44
    Recommendations   46

7. Action Through the Mass Media   52

    Representation of Health Issues in the Media   52
    Planned Use of the Media   54
    Recommendations   55

References and Suggested Further Reading   58

Appendix 1. World Health Organization Recommendations   59

Appendix 2. Example of a Regional Plan for the Prevention
            of Coronary Heart Disease   61

Appendix 3. Example of a District Plan for the Prevention
            of Coronary Heart Disease   73

Appendix 4. Action Guide — *So You Think You Want to Use
            the Media?*   81

Chapter One
INTRODUCTION

The Need for Action

Coronary heart disease in Britain kills more than 150,000 people each year — one person every three to four minutes. One man in 11 dies of a heart attack before he is 65 years old; and in at least an equal number the disease will have caused distressing symptoms, such as chest pain or shortness of breath. If such a problem had just arisen, there would be urgent calls for energetic action. But, perhaps because coronary heart disease has been around for some time, its inevitability has been widely accepted.

The costs are enormous, both human (through bereavement, disability and fear) and economic (by premature deaths and retirements, by sickness absence from work, and, increasingly, by demands on the medical services). Nor does there yet seem to be in this country the major decline in deaths from heart disease which is taking place in North America, Australia, Finland, Belgium, New Zealand, Norway and elsewhere.

The disease involves two underlying pathological processes. The first is atherosclerosis (hardening and narrowing of the arteries). This starts in childhood and ultimately affects nearly everyone, putting all at risk. By itself it is usually silent; but — often unpredictably — a second process may supervene, involving thrombosis (clotting) or other complications. At this stage death or manifest illness occurs. Both processes are amenable to prevention; but by the time symptoms develop, irreversible damage is likely to be present. The contribution of medical or surgical therapy is limited, both by the scale and by the nature of the problem. Prevention is essential. Prevention implies the correction of causes.

The familiar approach to the search for causes is to ask why some people become sick of a disease whilst others remain well. Applied to coronary heart disease this has identified the well-known 'risk factors', such as smoking, and the elevation of blood pressure and cholesterol. These personal characteristics focus concern on individuals, whose special risk reflects either their family background or features of their particular lifestyle. These susceptible people can be identified, and they require individual preventive advice.

There is another approach to the search for causes, and that is to ask not "*who* are the susceptible individuals?" but "*why* is this disease so common? *Why* is there an epidemic?". The answer to this question is to be found in characteristics of the population as a whole. Smoking and lack of exercise have come to be accepted as normal; and there is an increased risk even for those with *average* levels of blood cholesterol or blood pressure. Thus coronary heart disease has become a mass disease because of unhealthy characteristics of *average* life-style. This is a difficult concept, because it runs counter to the natural assumption that what most people do is alright. It points to a need for change in some widely accepted norms.

Historically the great successes of public health involved mass changes in the environment and in nutrition. The key to success lay in the fact that public authorities were able to regulate or supply the required changes, such as improved sanitation, clean air, and better quality of water and food. The prevention of coronary heart disease likewise calls for changes in supply, particularly in regard to food and cigarettes There are, however, two new features. The first is that the adoption of healthier habits (for example, of eating and exercise) calls for more active public participation and choice than did the acceptance of clean air and clean water: health education has become vital. The second is that whereas mass diseases of the past were linked with poverty, the emergence of mass coronary heart disease has coincided with prosperity. This does not mean that it is due to affluence *per se*. Indeed, it now bears more heavily on manual rather than professional workers, and its decline in various populations has occurred without a fall in living standards.

What requires to be changed is not affluence but only certain of its coincidental accompaniments. These include smoking, an unhealthy national diet and too little exercise (which also predisposes to obesity). Nevertheless, "with regard to several key preventive measures, the balance of evidence indicates sufficient assurance of safety and a sufficient probability of major benefits to warrant action at the population level. The evidence is similar in nature and strength to that governing past policy decisions on air pollution control, sanitary improvements, and the formulation of dietary requirements" (World Health Organization 1982). The scientific evidence, though extensive, does not amount to certain proof but is reasonable ground for energetic action.

The main aim with regard to action to prevent coronary heart disease should be reduction of its risk. Reduction of risk must not be equated with prevention, although the aim and hope is that this will occur.

The scientific basis for a policy on heart disease prevention has been reviewed in many authoritative reports, including the Joint Report by the Royal College of Physicians and the British Cardiac Society (1976). Despite a remarkable agreement in their main recommendations, little has been done to implement them. Concern at the absence of effective action led to the planning of the 'Canterbury Conference', on which this report is founded.

The Canterbury Conference and Report

The conference entitled 'Action to Prevent Coronary Heart Disease' discussed practical ways of implementing the major recommendations for reducing the incidence of coronary heart disease. (The scientific evidence for these recommendations had already been fully considered elsewhere.) This was the first time that such a wide-ranging discussion of the issues had been attempted.

A main reason for the absence of effective action in the United Kingdom has been the failure to bring together all the various interests and skills that are needed for implementation of existing proposals. These include – in addition to the providers of health services and their administrations – various government departments, the food industry and agricultural experts, economists, and experts in public education and the mass media.

Ultimately no fewer than 18 different disciplines were represented at the conference. Each of these disciplines is likely to be involved in any national programme to prevent coronary heart disease.

The Report on the Prevention of Coronary Heart Disease by an Expert Committee of the World Health Organization was selected as the basis for the conference discussions. This was because it was recent and authoritative, and it emphasised particularly the population approach to prevention. Its main recommendations are reproduced in Appendix 1.

The conference was sponsored by:

- The Health Education Council (who also funded the conference)
- The Department of Health and Social Security (in association with the health departments of Scotland, Northern Ireland and Wales)
- The British Cardiac Society
- The Coronary Prevention Group (who also gave administrative and secretarial support).

A wide range of other professional bodies agreed to be co-sponsors. These have been listed earlier together with the 80 conference participants and contributors. The sponsors and co-sponsors indicated their support for the general objectives of the conference, which were:

(i) To identify practical and efficient strategies for implementing in the United Kingdom the main recommendations of the 1982 WHO Expert Committee Report on the 'Prevention of Coronary Heart Disease'.

(ii) To examine the consequent implications for relevant areas of public policy.

The main conference discussions took place in six workshops each dealing with a major decision area: national policy, food and agriculture, Regional and District Health Authorities, primary health care, health education, and the mass media. The report follows the same plan. The workshop discussions centred around a major working document prepared for each in the preceding months by a small committee of experts. We are particularly grateful for the assistance of these committees and their convenors, as well as to the conference participants and chairmen. We also acknowledge the help of the Association of Area Medical Officers in initiating discussions about holding a conference.

After the conference the Steering Committee with the additional help of Don Nutbeam and Geoff Watts prepared an integrated report. This drew on the discussions at the conference and the summaries prepared by the individual workshops – as well as the pre-conference working documents and later work. A first draft was circulated to all participants. This final report was prepared in the light of their advice and comments, with valuable editorial assistance from John Catford and Christopher Robbins.

The planning of the conference and the authorship of the report were the responsibility of the Steering Committee. The contents therefore do not necessarily represent the views of sponsors, co-sponsors or individual participants.

The Canterbury Report offers a set of carefully considered proposals. Some are appropriate for action now, others are for continuing discussion and debate. Perhaps the main achievement of the conference so far has been the initiation of a dialogue between a wide range of people concerned about ways to reduce the burden of coronary heart disease. Future success of the conference now depends on the continuation of that dialogue so that there is effective and speedy ACTION TO PREVENT CORONARY HEART DISEASE.

Chapter Two
ACTION AT NATIONAL LEVEL

Policies aimed at preventing coronary heart disease concern many organisations and groups in addition to the National Health Service and the Health Education Council. The many factors which influence the main risks for coronary heart disease include smoking habits, the nation's diet, and exercise patterns in the community. Actions by the European Economic Community, the UK Government, manufacturing and service industries all affect the population's lifestyle through regulations, codes of practice, institutional policies, and economic and advertising pressures. A key task, therefore, is one of ensuring that the health implications of governmental and industrial actions are clearly recognised before decisions which might have an adverse effect on the risks for coronary heart disease are taken.

European Economic Community

The range of economic influences that affect the coronary risk factors are not easy to identify. They certainly include arrangements between Britain and the European Economic Community since one of the dominant influences on food supply is the Common Agricultural Policy. The way in which farm pricing policies affect the drive to produce foods of a particular type are especially important. The continuing problem of surplus milk and butter leads to pressures to subsidise these commodities and thereby promote an undesirably high consumption of fats rich in saturated acid. More indirect pressures also play a part since pricing policies on nitrogen fertilisers and cereal production affect the productivity of the dairy industry. Membership of the European Economic Community poses complex issues which are being tackled already for economic and political reasons. Nevertheless there are important health implications which also need to be considered when devising a long-term strategy for farming and other industries. A policy of relying on customer demand (for example for low fat products) to influence the economics of farming fails to anticipate farming needs and also neglects the way in which current policies affect the price of commodities and therefore their consumption. There is a need for the European Commission to recognise the importance of the consumer and the effects of policy changes on the population's health. Too often action is dominated by the short-term needs of the agricultural sector. Establishing on a European basis a consensus on the need for action to prevent coronary heart disease is of increasing importance and should be linked if possible to the growth of consumer interests. The role of the Ministry of Agriculture, Fisheries and Food in the European setting is discussed further in Chapter Three.

UK Government

Given the complex interaction of policies which affect lifestyles and hence coronary risk factors, it is important to consider how best the health implications of these can be heard effectively at a Central Governmental level. Many Ministerial responsibilities are already recognised and to some extent the Department of Health has links with other Ministries. For example, its Chief Medical Officer provides advice on health to the Ministry of Agriculture. Yet only comparatively recently has the need for vigorous preventive measures to combat the development of coronary heart disease been recognised in Britain. As a consequence, there is still considerable potential for improved inter-Departmental links and joint planning.

The Minister of Health and the Chief Medical Officer could be aided by a system which ensures that they have detailed analyses both of the health implications of possible economic measures and also of the cost of proposals aimed at preventing coronary heart disease. Both aspects are important because there is a range of preventive options which are likely to have different economic consequences. Economic analysis is therefore important. One method of ensuring an appropriate integration of issues relating to health would be to establish a Standing Committee in the Department of Health which could draw on contributions from the Treasury, and the Departments of Agriculture and Food, of Trade, and Industry and of Education and Science.

This proposal is suggested in preference to several others, including the establishment of a health orientated national body equivalent to a little 'NEDDY' (National Economic Development Office). A 'Health NEDDY' seems unlikely to succeed because there is little intrinsic economic advantage to the government, to business or to the trades union movement in such a proposal, despite the vast human benefits. A 'Health' seat on the 'NEDDY' itself, however, might be of benefit.

Development of a National Strategy

The World Health Organization in pursuing the goal of 'Health For All By The Year 2000' has called upon Member States to prepare national plans and programmes to implement policies to promote the health of their population. Great emphasis was also placed on this within the historic Declarations of Alma Ata in 1978 supported by the UK through the World Health Assembly and United Nations. The WHO European Regional Committee, on which the UK is also represented, is encouraging nations to develop a set of measurable targets as an integral part of a national health strategy.

The UK, as yet, has no national strategy for the promotion of health or the prevention of disease. As a result the tasks of the various organisations concerned have not been defined nor the rate of progress in achieving them stated. The National Health Service is no different in this respect. The situation here is in sharp contrast to some other western countries. The most notable example is the United States of America where in 1979 a national programme for improving the health of the American people entitled 'Healthy People' was published by the US Surgeon-General with Presidential support. In 1980, specific and measurable objectives were produced for 15 priority areas where action was necessary to achieve the health goals set for 1990.

There is an urgent need for the British Government through the Department of Health to formulate national policies and programmes for health promotion and disease prevention. The prevention of coronary heart disease would be an important integral part of such a strategy, and this would enable co-ordinated action on a wide front. The succeeding chapters describe detailed ways in which progress could be made. Their effectiveness would be greatly improved if they were part of an agreed national programme in which all agencies worked together in a comprehensive and supportive way. It is clear that national leadership and planning are required over and above the general policy guidelines that have come from central government so far.

National Organisations

The National Health Service and the Health Education Council clearly have a major role to play in the prevention of coronary heart disease. Their contributions are considered in detail in Chapters Four, Five and Six. Central government will need to ensure that adequate resources are made available so that real progress is made. Leadership from the Departments of Health is vital.

The part that the food and agricultural industries can play is discussed in Chapter Three, and in this field the Ministry of Agriculture, Fisheries and Food will be able to make a major contribution. The Department of Education and Science does much and could do more to promote improved health education in schools, as outlined in Chapter Six. The Department of Trade and Industry will also need to plan constructively so that those industries manufacturing or distributing tobacco products can diversify, in view of the expected widespread decline in tobacco sales.

Many other organisations at national and local level have a part to play. For example, the Confederation of British Industry and the trades union movement, together with the Health and Safety Executive could do much to promote the health of their staff and members. Many neglected areas of provision within industry would become apparent if businesses published statements on the welfare of their workers as part of their annual reports.

This could lead to action concerning catering arrangements, occupational health services, provision of non-smoking areas and exercise facilities. The Sports Council and Local Authority Recreation Departments could also lend their support in raising the level of physical activity within the community, particularly amongst groups that take little exercise. Programmes should link particularly with the Sports Council's national plan for young people and middle-aged 'Sport in the Community: the next 10 years'. A National Fitness Survey, physiological and behavioural, would be an essential element, to generate public interest and enthusiasm and as a baseline for monitoring progress.

Chapter Five on action within primary health care emphasises that preventive approaches are often different to those concerning the diagnosis and management of illness. There is a need then to ensure that health professionals have sufficient skills and information to contribute to prevention. This will not be achieved unless there are effective teachers working at undergraduate, postgraduate, and continuing education levels.

Professional bodies such as the Royal Colleges have a responsibility for training and education as well as ensuring high standards of professional competence. They should ensure that national policies for teaching prevention are developed in medical, dental and nursing schools.

Ginger groups such as ASH (Action on Smoking and Health) and the Coronary Prevention Group have played a useful role in raising public awareness of the important health issues. Their contribution needs to be strengthened. Health charities such as the British Heart Foundation and the Chest, Heart and Stroke Association and other voluntary organisations also have much to offer. However the UK, unlike several other developed countries, lacks an active authoritative body at national level to speak out for policies directed at the prevention of coronary heart disease. Some of the progress in Australia, Finland and the United States has been attributed to the activities of their respective Heart Associations. This deficiency needs to be addressed as a matter of urgency.

Controlling the Smoking Epidemic

Action to reduce the high levels of smoking in the UK is a vital part of any programme of coronary heart disease prevention, and this is a recurrent theme throughout the report. The prevention of smoking has long been the concern of the Royal College of Physicians and their most recent report published in 1983 outlines a comprehensive range of actions. It is not necessary, therefore, to repeat these recommendations but to highlight those of national significance.

The smoking message needs to be uncompromising; it is total abstention. There is no evidence that any one type of cigarette is less likely than another to cause coronary heart disease. Product alteration is unlikely, therefore, to have an impact, and the promotion of a so-called 'safer' cigarette could actually be counter-productive in giving smokers a false sense of assurance.

The price of tobacco is known to influence its sale, and a progressive increase in tax to ensure that the cost of tobacco rises faster than the rate of inflation is an important fiscal measure to influence smoking in the short term.

Of great concern is the fate of children and young adults who still remain susceptible to promotion of tobacco and peer pressures. Alarming numbers of children are still taking up smoking despite substantial efforts to improve health education and widespread recognition of the major health hazards of smoking. There should, therefore, be a ban on the sales promotion of tobacco as well as on sports sponsorship which associates smoking with healthy activities. Since voluntary agreements with the industry are insufficient, legislation should be introduced to control advertising, promotion, etc. Mandatory warning notices on cigarette packets should be more prominent and stronger.

The continuing sales of tobacco to under-age children is very worrying. This practice can only be blocked effectively if tobacconists, like publicans, are licensed before they are eligible to sell cigarettes to adults. To lose their licence for illegal sales to children would then constitute a serious deterrent. The shops themselves should also have a large health warning prominently displayed on their door so that there is no doubt in the public's mind of the healthier way of life of non-smokers.

Recommendations

1. A national strategy for the prevention of coronary heart disease should be established, preferably as part of a comprehensive strategy for the promotion of health and the prevention of disease.

This should be formulated by central government, through the Department of Health, in consultation with all the various agencies and organisations concerned. It should state the various contributions expected including that of government departments and industry. Objectives and targets will need to be set and their achievements carefully monitored. Programmes will need to be carefully costed and when agreed, real resources will need to be made available.

2. The Department of Health should advance the prevention of coronary heart disease to become a major priority for itself and the National Health Service. There are existing mechanisms, such as through the planning system and review procedures, for pursuing this aim and these should be activated.

3. A standing committee should be established within the Department of Health to review all economic and other policies which have a bearing on health and in particular coronary heart disease. Improved working relationships need to be developed with other government departments so that they accept fuller responsibility for improving the health as well as the wealth of the nation.

4. A seat should be available on the National Economic Development Council (NEDDY) for a health representative so that the health consequences of economic policies can be fully considered.

5. The recent recommendations of the Royal College of Physicians on the prevention and control of smoking should be implemented. There should be no attempt to promote the consumption of so-called 'safer' cigarettes.

6. The health implications for food policy should be discussed more widely, both in the UK and in the European Economic Community, through the European Parliament and Commission. The aim would be to establish a consensus on the need for action to prevent coronary heart disease.

7. The Secretary of State for Agriculture, Fisheries and Food should promote the inclusion of health issues in the development of food policy both in the UK, and in Europe through the Food Directorate in Brussels. This would be in addition to the current activities relating to the legalistic aspects of labelling, additives, etc.

8. Existing agencies, such as the Royal Colleges, the British Cardiac Society, the British Heart Foundation, the Coronary Prevention Group, the Health Education Council and the DHSS, should promote the cause of coronary heart disease prevention. To this end, it is recommended that they should form a working party

to discuss as a matter of urgency how progress might be made — particularly at a national level.

9. Professional bodies, universities and training colleges have a major responsibility to ensure that both health and education professionals are appropriately trained in prevention. Urgent attention should be given to pre- and post-qualification teaching and in-service training.

10. Other national organisations such as the Confederation of British Industry (CBI), trades union movement, Sports Council, health charities and voluntary organisations, should lend their active support to the pursuit of prevention.

11. A National Fitness Survey should be established to complement those monitoring activities at national level concerning smoking (by the Office of Population Censuses and Surveys) and diet (by the Ministry of Agriculture, Fisheries and Food).

Chapter Three
ACTION WITHIN THE FOOD AND AGRICULTURAL INDUSTRIES

The agricultural and food industries can make a major contribution to implementing the recommendations of the World Health Organization to reduce the average intake of fat (especially saturated fat), sugar and salt and to increase the intake of dietary fibre. However, the specific targets proposed by the World Health Organization are of an ideal or long-term nature. Intermediate targets are required which would gain wider acceptance and which could be achieved within the next decade.

Progressive adjustments to the types of food produced can then be matched with an increase in the awareness and knowledge of nutritional factors and health in consumers. A move toward healthier eating patterns can therefore be seen as occurring in two ways: either as a change from above or as change from below.

Change from above happens when policy initiatives whether of Government (e.g. the Ministry of Agriculture, Fisheries and Food — MAFF) or of the relevant food industries, affect the overall composition of food. A wide range of policies can be involved in this process.

Change from below, on the other hand, can occur through increasing awareness and the changing attitudes of consumers in food selection and in healthier eating. While change from below cannot be totally separated from change from above, this chapter is concerned with the potential for, and implications of, change in policy affecting food supply. Chapters Four to Seven cover the consumer, education and information aspects in detail.

Dietary Goals for Agriculture

The development of dietary goals or guidelines can be helpful to the agricultural and food industries because they provide a clear indication of the nature and extent of change suggested on scientific and health grounds by health professionals. The development of these 'goals' is not the responsibility of the agricultural and food industries, nor indeed of MAFF. MAFF and the food industry can together modify the nature of the foodstuffs entering the distribution chain. They can thereby exert a more powerful effect in relation to the population problem of coronary heart disease than can be achieved by the patient-orientated approach of the health services. Nevertheless MAFF is not the appropriate Government agency to initiate such a programme. This programme should be defined by the Department of Health in terms of dietary goals for the population which MAFF would then implement within an overall food and health policy. Once the goals are set it could then be helpful to have the Parliamentary Select Committee on Agriculture examine the most effective ways of implementing change and thereby ensure as wide agreement as possible for the actions needed.

This logical distribution of responsibility between the Department of Health, MAFF and industry has, however, to be seen in the context of the British agriculture and food industries. To advocate too rapid a change could be counter-productive and might generate unnecessary opposition. This is why quantified long-term targets should not be offered initially. Rather it would be more effective to propose interim targets such as those advocated by the National Advisory Committee for Nutrition Education (NACNE). The NACNE targets could be updated in a rolling programme which takes into account new research and the lessons from implementation.

This practical approach is important because implementation by the UK of the full World Health Organization's recommendations would involve major reductions in the farm output of meat, fat, milk and butter. Some of these changes are likely to be needed in any case as

TABLE I. The degree of self-sufficiency* in Europe and the UK: 1979-80

	EEC (inc. UK) %	UK %
Soft wheat	114	77
Hard wheat	91	–
Barley	111	114
Oats	96	91
Grain maize	62	–
Potatoes	101	95
Sugar	125	48
Vegetables	?	74
Fresh fruit	?	32
Wine	112	–
Vegetable fats and oils	?	11
Skimmed milk powder	135	329
Cheese	104	72
Butter	120	51
Eggs	101	98

Source: Eurostat (1982)

* The self-sufficiency level is a ratio (expressed as a percentage) of the domestic production of a food to the domestic production, plus total imports but minus any exports. It is a measure of the proportion of the total usage of a food which is produced in the UK.

part of a rationalisation of the Common Agricultural Policy. To advocate them in full at present gives the misleading impression that nationally we should enforce rapid and extensive changes on the agricultural industry. The degree of self-sufficiency in Britain and the European Economic Community for the principal products of concern is given in Table I, indicating that some reductions could occur in consumption without damaging the British agricultural industry.

The changes being proposed here in the British diet do not threaten the overall security of the food and agricultural industries, since people will continue to eat food. They do, however, imply a substantial redistribution of food preferences and a shift in the compositon of diets. But we do not doubt the ability of the production and marketing systems to adapt successfully to the changes, given time and intelligent anticipation.

As long as the whole industry is involved, these changes should be welcomed as reinforcing some of the trends towards 'healthier' products already apparent in the increased production of wholemeal breads, spreads low in saturated fat etc and innovations such as low-salt bacon.

Ministry of Agriculture, Fisheries and Food

The importance of the Common Agricultural Policy has already been mentioned in discussions of national policy (Chapter Two). Some of MAFF's actions, particularly in relation to intake of animal fats and sugars, are limited by membership of the European Economic Community. The present operation of the Common Agricultural Policy in relation to dairy products and sugar is directly opposed to the food and health policy the UK should be aiming for.

MAFF should ensure, therefore, that health aspects are taken more fully into account during the major remodelling of the Policy that is likely to take place over the next few years. Thus the Community's proposals to raise the prescribed fat content of milk should be opposed. The present consumer subsidy on butter should be removed, and the Community should phase out the purchase of skimmed milk under its intervention programme since this acts as a hidden subsidy on butter production. Import levies on oilseeds and vegetable oils should also be opposed.

An important feature of the UK food chain is that at least 75 per cent of food is processed or manufactured before it reaches the consumer; thus if MAFF can work effectively with the food processing industry it can profoundly affect most of the food entering consumption. MAFF already has the responsibility for ensuring that all foods are safe and wholesome. Historically several legislative constraints have been placed on the food industry, but legislation has the disadvantage of being cumbersome and inflexible. For example, it is difficult to amend in 1988 a standard defined by statute in 1984. Legislation also tends to reduce the co-operation of the interested groups, whereas the aim should be to develop a positive policy of co-operation with the food industry so that a food and health policy works.

To overcome these problems it is customary to develop codes of practice. These have the advantage that (a) the food industry is seen to play a positive role in drawing up the codes, and (b) the codes can be regularly updated to accommodate the rolling targets foreseen in the later stages of the programme. Clearly, should the codes fail to be effective there would then be the option of returning to the legislative mechanism.

On the basis of codes of practice we envisage MAFF and the food industry, with continuing support from DHSS, setting the industry a series of targets aiming at a steady reduction in the amounts of saturated fat, sugar and salt entering the UK diet via processed foods. This would not mean a *pro rata* reduction in all foods, and the involvement of the industry would be essential to ensure getting the optimum market mix. MAFF already operates the National Food Survey. This, with some modification and complemented by information on food consumed outside the home, would be an effective way of monitoring the progress of the proposed programme.

MAFF should also be responsible for encouraging changes in agricultural production which would be consistent with, and necessary to the new requirements of the processing sector. However, MAFF often cannot act independently of the Common Agricultural Policy. For example, there is a requirement for a degree of fatness in cattle and sheep before subsidy is paid, which leads to more fat than necessary entering the meat chain. MAFF should act to reduce this. However, a change in grading standards for carcasses would be an important step which the UK could implement directly.

MAFF should closely examine existing food regulations to bring them into line with the agreed nutritional objectives. Some existing regulations could hamper the proposed dietary changes, e.g. the present minimal requirement for sugar in sugar-containing soft drinks, and the limitations on vegetable protein in sausages. It would also be important to examine codes of practice and existing legislation affecting description and labelling of foods, which must be informative enough to allow the consumer to select intelligently from the range of foods that will continue to be marketed. Thus while we envisage a gradual reduction in the fat content of all sausages, high, medium and low fat brands will continue to be available. These should be clearly and simply labelled, e.g. using a 'traffic light' system.

Consumer Attitudes and Needs

Although the dietary changes proposed are gradual, they could fairly quickly lead to changes in consumption of some foods once they are perceived by consumers to have been altered to conform with modern nutritional views. Since an essential part of the Strategy is that consumer demand should also gradually change in phase with the changes in food entering the food chain, more needs to be known about consumer perception of 'food quality'. This is over and above the wider awareness of 'healthy' food that will be stimulated by health educators, etc. This should not be done by the food industry itself, as this could be confounded by marketing strategies of individual companies. MAFF might like to consider, therefore, sponsoring a clearly defined study by the Social Science Research Council.

Consumer demand for healthier products could also be stimulated by the food industry. It is important that products such as low-fat milk should be universally available. Commercial advertising, as well as that of the Health Education Council, has an important role. If the food industry as a whole were co-operating in the overall strategy for food and health, its advertising would be likely to mirror and encourage the dietary changes being sought. However, it must be recognised that some advertising could run counter to the main objective. If this appeared significant, then a system for regulating advertising, preferably through existing bodies, would be needed to ensure that it did not promote unhealthy or misleading information – as has already been accepted in the case of slimming foods.

The range of outlets for 'healthy' foods should be extended (e.g. by supply of low fat milk by milk roundsmen and schools, options which are not at present encouraged). Food and health policies at a District level should in particular seek to involve local retail outlets in their health promotion programmes, perhaps through local Chambers of Commerce.

Whilst the main initiatives in implementing this dietary programme need to be taken by MAFF, the Department of Education and Science could play an important part. The Department could give powerful support by developing a more nutritionally sound school meals programme. It could insist on the inclusion of the concepts of nutrition and health in a wide range of classroom activities and not just by having 'special' lessons on nutrition and health. School children would then be widely exposed to the concept that what they eat is important to their future health.

Consumer responsiveness to health education is unlikely to proceed effectively without food labelling of a simple type. The danger of the present position is that as consumer pressure for more specific health education grows, those involved in offering advice will be forced to suggest changes in dietary selection which exclude a range of food products from the diet. This might then lead to general acceptance of the idea that 'convenience' and 'processed' foods are intrinsically unhealthy and be counter-productive to the promotion of appropriately constituted foods developed by the food manufacturing industries.

At present it is very difficult for consumers to make simple and rapid choices if they seek to purchase foods which are lower in sugar, fat and salt content. The time has now come for a careful study of the most effective way of presenting food composition on labels. Improvements in food labelling would allow the consumer greater choice of foods and the opportunity to exercise some personal influence on the dietary prevention of coronary heart disease.

Research and Development

This chapter has started to consider some of the possible effects of the proposed measures on the UK agricultural industry, but more research and analysis is required. Agriculture has been developed as a high input/high output industry, with much of that output in the dairy products, animal fat and sugar sectors, for which reduced consumption is proposed. Urgent attention should now be given to the technological and economic aspects of alternative lower input/lower output systems. These should aim at maintaining rural populations and prosperity, despite a reduction in output of certain products, particularly milk.

Increased research and development effort should also be given to the more rapid reduction of the fat content of meat animals. Other sectors of agriculture could make a considerable impact on the fat being produced during livestock production.

More research and development is also needed in the food/nutrition/health interfaces. As the heart disease prevention programme develops, progressive changes in diet can then be proposed in response to a better understanding of metabolic pathways and the role of nutrition. The health properties of the food produced by UK agriculture, and of the processing of that food, should be an important part of the remit of the Board and Committees of the Joint Consultative Organisation. Health considerations could then influence their advice to government departments on priorities for research and development in agriculture and food.

Recommendations

1. A practical national food and health policy should be formulated by the Department of Health to provide national, quantified dietary

goals and guidelines as a basis for policy implementation by the Ministry of Agriculture, Fisheries and Food (MAFF). A rolling programme of changes based, for example, initially on the interim targets of NACNE would permit achievable objectives to be set without alienating the agricultural and food sectors of industry.

2. The Parliamentary Select Committee on Agriculture should be invited to examine the most effective ways of implementing the national dietary goals with particular emphasis on accommodating the diverse views and interests of those who would be involved in changes in the food supply.

3. Ministers and MAFF should oppose those elements of the Common Agricultural Policy which run counter to a healthy food policy. (See also Chapter One recommendations 6, 7.)

4. MAFF could consider the following ways of reducing the fat, sugar and salt content of the national food supply:

    (i)   Adjusting the carcass grading systems for sheep, cattle and pigs to encourage farmers by incentives to produce lean carcasses.

    (ii) Examining and altering existing food regulations to provide opportunities for manufacturers to improve food composition and make foods compatible with nutritional objectives.

    (iii) Shifting subsidy support for agriculture away from milk, fat and sugar production towards sectors of agriculture which can make a positive contribution to a more healthy diet, e.g. potatoes, fish, vegetables and fruit, bread-making wheat.

5. Codes of practice should be drawn up by MAFF and the food industry which set a series of targets aiming at a steady reduction in the amounts of saturated fat, sugar and salt entering the UK diet via processed foods. Reducing the content of these substances in meat products, milk, breakfast cereals, tinned foods, biscuits and cakes etc presents opportunities for industrial innovation and sales promotion.

6. Food labelling should be improved as a matter of urgency. This may be achieved through voluntary codes of practice which allow greater flexibility without the need for additional legislation. Labelling needs to be consumer-orientated and hence clear and simple. A 'traffic light' system should be investigated.

7. Since advertising and marketing can exert an important influence on a healthier eating practice, codes of practice should be agreed. These should allow flexible and early improvements in agricultural practice.

8. Attention should be given to the development of lower input/
   lower output technologies and production systems in agriculture.
   Changes would need to encompass economic difficulties, and to
   contribute to rural population maintenance and prosperity. Research
   and development should also be directed to methods for reducing
   carcass fat content and perhaps for changing the fatty acid composition of dairy fat.

9. Much more research is needed into the most effective ways of
   reducing diet-related disease. Research and development programmes within industry should take full cognisance of the general
   policy shift towards healthier foods.

10. The 'health' properties of the food produced by UK agriculture,
    and of the processing of that food, should be an important part of
    the remit of the Board and Committees of the Joint Consultative
    Organisation. These would then influence their advice to the
    Ministry of Agriculture, Fisheries and Food; Department of Agri-
    culture and Fisheries for Scotland; the Department of Agriculture
    for Northern Ireland; the Agricultural and Food Research Council;
    and other bodies on research and development priorities.

11. Wider consumer representation on the Food Advisory Committee
    should be sought, and the basis for the Committee's deliberations
    and its conclusions should be more freely available to health workers
    and to the public.

12. The range of outlets for 'healthy' foods should be extended, e.g.
    supply of low fat milk by roundsmen and in schools. Such products
    need to be priced competitively.

13. The Department of Education and Science should reconsider the
    role of schools in developing a better understanding of nutrition
    and health in children. The diverse arrangements for school meals
    need to be reassessed. The Home Economics classroom and the
    dining room should provide examples of attractive and nutrition-
    ally appropriate meals.

Chapter Four
ACTION THROUGH THE NATIONAL HEALTH SERVICE

Within the National Health Service (NHS) the prevention of coronary heart disease needs to be considered alongside other areas of health promotion and disease prevention. Action directed at smoking, unhealthy nutrition, physical inactivity and hypertension will have a major impact on many other important causes of ill-health in Britain today. Valuable benefits will be expected in the prevention of stroke, cancer, respiratory disease, mental and physical handicap, perinatal mortality, dental disease and psychiatric disorders, as well as enhancing a sense of wellbeing. The actions to be considered, therefore, for the prevention of coronary heart disease will help to promote the total health of the nation.

Role of the National Health Service

Regional and District Health Authorities have a crucial role to play in the prevention of coronary heart disease. They have a statutory obligation which is clearly concerned with enhancing the health of their population. Importantly, each Authority has the organisational framework and professional resources to fulfil that obligation. In the majority of health authorities this responsibility has not been accepted, nor the potential realised. Inadequate resources have therefore been made available by them for the prevention of coronary heart disease.

There are two integrated approaches which are seen to be cornerstones of health authority strategies — one involving the whole population, the other targeting high risk groups. Primary care teams and health education departments, supported by other health professionals, offer the greatest contribution from the National Health Service towards the prevention of coronary heart disease. The task of Regional and District planning is to provide stimulation and support to these activities.

Whilst acknowledging the influence of local options, it is clear that health authority policies and programmes are to a large extent governed by nationally determined priorities. If the National Health Service is to respond in an effective way, a national 'push' will be required, needing a comprehensive and integrated national strategy. Such a national plan will need to indicate the contributions that will be made by the variety of other agencies, outside the National Health Service, that influence health. The US document 'Objectives for the Nation' (1980) as a sequel to 'Healthy People' (1979), which was mentioned in Chapter Two, is an example of what can be achieved.

Development of Planning and Monitoring

Within the NHS, Regional and District Authorities are already required to produce 10-year strategic and annual operational plans with a strategy review every five years. Health promotion and disease prevention policies and programmes, particularly for heart disease, should receive a high and specifically quantified priority.

Unlike some other countries, Britain lacks a database at Regional and District level to monitor changes in risk factors for heart disease. There is currently inadequate information available on published statements of District and Regional health promotion policies, priorities, targets, and timed and costed programmes.

The Accountability Reviews introduced by the Secretary of State in 1982 are designed to enforce accountability by the NHS for the implementation of nationally and locally predetermined objectives. Whilst the full impact of this review process has yet to emerge, it is nevertheless a potentially strong mechanism for use in conjunction with the planning system for developing and implementing strategies for the prevention of heart disease and for providing the necessary information to monitor progress.

The NHS planning system in conjunction with the less formalised but potentially powerful mechanisms available to the DHSS could be used to:

- establish policies and programmes
- direct resources
- provide for the setting up of organisational structures, which are necessary to generate commitment, and implement and evaluate programmes.

The Health Education Council can provide much needed support to health authorities in the fields of mass media intervention (i.e. marketing techniques) and training. However, lack of 'regionalisation' of the Council's activities has meant that in the past few programmes have been jointly planned with health authorities to achieve the greatest effect.

Importance of Local Input

Regional and District planning for coronary heart disease prevention will inevitably focus on the formal managerial process, but this is not enough. Health authorities must be sensitive to the need to secure local community and professional participation in policy development and implementation. This will promote strong commitment to action and a sensitivity to local organisational and environmental needs and possibilities.

Neighbourhood health strategies and programmes are crucial to grassroots progress. There is a need for special initiatives to develop or to use existing neighbourhood groups to integrate both professional and community effort. Health could thus be promoted within the wider context of community development. Health workers concerned with encouraging and supporting community action and Primary Health Care Team involvement are therefore particularly important. (See also Chapters Four and Six.)

Example or 'model' plans could help discussion at Regional and District level once initial commitment to action has been obtained. However, it needs to be emphasised that they should not be seen as prescriptive and will inevitably be modified and elaborated to meet local circumstances.

Funding Sources and Mechanisms

A stable resource base for coronary heart disease prevention will be necessary to secure widespread progress. In view of current NHS resourcing problems and the relatively fixed pattern of funding to meet operational health-care commitments, progress is unlikely to be achieved except through an initial centrally-funded pump-priming initiative for at least three to five years.

Central funding, crucially important though it is, is not the only available resource. Authorities should review the use of existing resources and professional skills, for example NHS training and community health service budgets. There are also other sources of funds:

- joint financing, particularly for community-based programmes
- inner-city Partnership monies and other special funds to particular authorities
- youth employment programmes, and
- non-recurring resources, often available every year arising from the 'bank-rolling' of revenue developments for forthcoming capital programmes and general under-spending due to slippage of such programmes.

Authorities should be more opportunistic in their approach to funding prevention programmes.

Recommendations

1. **National and Government Level**

(i) A national strategy for the prevention of coronary heart disease should be formulated by central government with clearly defined objectives and targets. The role that the NHS will be expected to play should be explicitly stated and the mechanisms determined by which the Department of Health will ensure that quantified progress is made. The responsibilities of other agencies that influence health should be recognised, and the particular tasks that they will undertake to support the Strategy should be identified.

(ii) Prevention of coronary heart disease should be incorporated into the formal NHS planning system and accountability review process. Chairmen of Regional Health Authorities should emphasise the importance of this during their discussions with the Secretary of State and Health Ministers.

(iii) Pump-priming grants for a five-year period should be available to Regions and Districts to initiate heart disease prevention programmes. The Department of Health should announce the initiative 12 months before the grants are available to ensure full discussion and proper planning at District, Unit, Primary Care Team and Community level. It is recommended that a minimum of £30,000 per annum should be available to Regional Health Authorities to establish their regional role, together with a sum for use by Districts calculated on the basis of a minimum of 20p per head of total population per annum. Districts would be eligible to claim these funds from the Region on the production of timed and costed programmes. The total cost of such an initiative would therefore amount to £9.7 million per annum for the English Regions, and approximately £12 million per annum for the whole UK.

(iv) The Health Education Council and Scottish Health Education Group should spend a minimum of 10p per head of total population per annum on mass media initiatives, jointly planned with Regions and Districts. To be effective this will require regionalisation of the Council's initiatives with the establishment of Regional planning and operational teams of perhaps two to three persons per Region. These organisations will also need to sponsor additional training and research. They are in the best position to calculate the total increase in their budgets and staffing required to meet these developments. The English Regions will need, therefore, a mass media budget of £5 million per annum, a training and research budget of £0.5 million per annum, and an increase in staffing of around 40 posts to meet the needs of the Regional planning and operational teams. Overall at least £8 million per annum will be required for the UK.

(v) Greater emphasis needs to be placed on the monitoring of progress in heart disease prevention. Simple, low cost methods of measuring changes in the prevalence of risk factors at Regional, District and Primary Care Team level are required. The DHSS and the Health Education Council should commission as a matter of urgency a detailed review of the progress already made in this field by some other countries (e.g. Australia, Canada, Finland and the United States). Following such a review, pilot studies should be undertaken to develop UK equivalents of measures of performance and tools to facilitate periodic monitoring. These would also provide a lead to the rest of the service in search for indicators of effectiveness.

(vi) At national and local government level, chairmen, members and chief officers should recognise their responsibilities and opportunities to press for wider kinds of improvements which will promote healthy lifestyles.

They should systematically seek, for example, at local government level:

(a)   To obtain the participation in public education programmes of teachers, youth workers, social workers, community development workers, home helps, recreation centre staff and other staff in regular contact with the public.

(b)   To obtain support of environmental health officers in encouraging employers, whom they visit, to implement health promotion policies concerning non-smoking, healthy eating and exercise, including the provision of appropriate facilities.

(c)   To improve nutrition in schools, local authority workplaces and residential and day care accommodation.

(d)   To extend non-smoking areas in local authority workplaces and public buildings.

(e)   To provide more community facilities for exercise and recreation and especially to make school facilities more widely available outside normal school hours.

and at national level:

(f)   To strengthen the Health Education Council and to develop better mechanisms for joint planning along the lines discussed above, whilst recognising its important contribution to date.

(g) To increase taxation on tobacco to discourage consumption.

(h) To ban all cigarette advertising, including sport and arts sponsorship.

(i) To achieve food labelling, especially regarding the energy fat (and type of fat) and salt content of manufactured foods.

(j) To secure a progressive reduction in the fat and salt content of manufactured food.

(k) To obtain tax incentives for employers who provide exercise facilities for employees and families.

(l) To encourage distribution of healthy food products which are accessible to all and competitively priced, e.g. fresh pasteurised skimmed milk, wholemeal bread.

(m) To encourage lower cost life insurance, etc, for those with healthy lifestyles.

2. Regional Health Authority Level

(i) Within the NHS planning system and following full consultation with District Health Authorities and uses of the advisory machinery, Regional Health Authorities should publish a plan on the prevention of coronary heart disease. This should ideally be part of a wider Regional Plan on the promotion of health and the prevention of disease. The plan should contain:

(a) A health goal, which should indicate the scale of improvement that is sought in terms of a reduction of premature death rates from coronary heart disease over a 10-year period. Such a calculation should be based on the experience of similar western countries where reductions have occurred. The planned reduction in deaths should be given as an informative reference point for the general community.

(b) Specific objectives whereby this goal is sought to be achieved, and primary and secondary target levels of achievement for the next five and 10 years. Primary targets would refer to changes in the lifestyles hazardous to health, e.g. smoking. Secondary targets would refer to levels of activity, including programmes and infrastructure considered to be necessary to achieve the primary target levels. Failure to achieve the set targets would indicate the need to reconsider policies, programmes and resources.

(c) Details of preventive programmes to be undertaken directly
by the Regional Health Authority.

(d) Details or guidelines which District Health Authorities will
be required to follow in drawing up planning proposals.

(e) An outline of resource assumptions and funding mechanisms
for the planning period which Authorities will need in order
to plan within realistic resource expectations.

(f) Details of the infrastructure at Regional level required to
implement the policy.

(g) A report of the progress made to date and the method by
which future progress will be monitored and quantified.

(ii) A small interdisciplinary advisory or 'ginger group' should be
established in each Region made up of enthusiastic and committed
officers and health care professionals with the terms of reference
broadly defined in Appendix 2. This would also include Health
Education Council staff specially designated to develop initiatives
in the Region. The group should co-ordinate regionwide effort,
provide support, monitor progress and act as a catalyst. This should
ideally be a sub-group of a Regional Health Promotion Group, which
has a comprehensive brief for health promotion and disease prevention in the Region.

(iii) The post of a Regional Health Promotion Officer with special
responsibilities for heart disease prevention should be established
to provide executive and professional support for the advisory
group. It is proposed that discussions be held with the Health
Education Council to explore the potential for joint funding of
such posts to ensure joint planning of programmes.

(iv) An information base covering the prevalence of risk factors and
levels of knowledge and attitudes in the community should be
obtained. Such data are of key importance. Together with the
setting of realistic targets for particular programmes, better information will help achieve maximum progress in heart disease prevention. Monitoring programmes will require careful planning
with technical support from Regional statistical and information
departments.

(v) The Regional role in postgraduate education and training, together
with District support for in-service training and induction programmes, should be reconsidered so that maximum support can be
given to preventive programmes. The potential contribution from
existing staff employed within other divisions of the Regional

Health Authorities, e.g. press and public relations should also be reviewed.

3. District Health Authority Level

(i) Within the NHS planning system, and following full consultation with health professionals and the community, District Health Authorities should publish their plans on the prevention of coronary heart disease.

These should contain details of:

(a) The infrastructure required to implement the Plan.

(b) The mechanism whereby resources will be made available for heart disease prevention and a description of those resources.

(c) The method by which the active participation and support of the following will be obtained:

● general practitioners
● clinicians
● local authorities
● community groups
● voluntary organisations.

(d) The part that the District Health Education Service will play.

(e) The part that the community health services, and in particular health visitors, will play.

(f) Details of District policy and programmes directed at:

● the prevention and cessation of smoking
● the promotion of healthy nutrition
● the promotion of sensible exercise
● the control of hypertension.

(g) Reports on progress to date and the methods by which progress will be monitored in the future, so that modifications to programmes can be made if required.

(ii) Interdisciplinary Heart Disease Prevention Teams should be set up in each District, with the constitution and terms of reference broadly described in Appendix 3. They will help with formulation, steering and co-ordination of programmes. However, they cannot hope to have the sensitivity to specific local needs and possibilities for action that more informal and locally based teams will have.

If properly constituted with senior membership, they should be able to make progress managerially and politically. Sub-groups will be required, for example, for developing health education policy and programmes (see Chapter Six).

(iii) Neighbourhood health promotion groups are recommended, using health or community centres as a focal point for joint professional and community interaction. These groups, together with other interest groups, would provide a more sensitive framework for local planning, commitment and action. They will need financial support from Authorities, often on a one-off basis.

(iv) The appointment of an additional Health Education/Promotion Officer to develop community action is strongly commended as part of an essential expansion of District Health Education/Promotion resources, to facilitate and stimulate neighbourhood groups. (See also Chapter Six.) In addition, there needs to be an energetic but acceptable Primary Care Team liaison person to facilitate and stimulate action within the Primary Care Teams in the District. (See also Chapters Five and Six.) Such an appointment could be adequately filled by a general practitioner employed on a sessional basis by the health authority.

(v) The NHS itself is a community. Emphasis needs to be given to the contribution that health service management and the Occupational Health Service can make to the achievement of established targets by NHS employees themselves. Reductions in risk factors amongst NHS employees should precede those in the general population in view of:

(a)   The relative ease of implementing programmes for a defined population within the NHS.

(b)   The important exemplar role of NHS staff in the community and their potential as health educators.

Specific programmes for heart disease prevention need to be developed for NHS staff and carefully monitored. Organisational changes are likely to be required to support the programmes, e.g. provision of no-smoking areas, exercise facilities and changing rooms, and healthy nutrition.

(vi) In addition to pump-priming grants from the Department of Health and the Regional Health Authority, Districts should consider other ways of obtaining resources for heart disease prevention programmes, such as through:

(a)   Realignment of the work of hospital and community health staff especially health visitors.

(b)   Joint finance.

(c)   Non-recurring monies, e.g. from capital programmes slippage or stored revenue to meet the consequences of future programmes.

(d)   Inner-city partnership monies and other special funds to local authorities.

(e)   Youth employment programmes.

(f)   Charities and local firms and employers.

Although short-term funding will be helpful to initiate programmes, longer term planning needs to be commenced forthwith. This might seek to expand, for example, health visitor and health education services, so that heart disease prevention activities can be sustained on a stable resource base.

4. Implementation of programmes

(i)   Discussion should start at once at Regional and District level about the need to mount an ambitious and energetic programme directed at coronary heart disease prevention. All appropriate professional groups should be included as well as the community itself. Attractive and accessible educational programmes (seminars, conferences, study days, etc) should be mounted to facilitate this.

(ii)   At a suitable point in these discussions, the example or 'model' Regional and District plans contained in Appendices 2 and 3 should be presented. It should be emphasised at meetings and in documents that these are not prescriptive and will need to be modified and elaborated to meet local circumstances.

(iii) It is imperative that Regions and Districts should move sufficiently quickly over the next 12 months so that an outline strategy for heart disease prevention is included in the next quinquennial/decennial NHS Strategy development process. Regional and District Strategies for the next 10 years will be finalised and published in March 1985. Prevention is one of the topics to be included, and there is therefore an ideal opportunity for heart disease prevention measures to be identified so that as resources become available action can commence during the subsequent years.

Chapter Five
ACTION WITHIN PRIMARY HEALTH CARE

This chapter proposes ways in which the Primary Health Care Team can play a full part in preventing coronary heart disease. These focus on identifying what the Team can contribute and how Team members might be encouraged to act. Reports on prevention published by the Royal College of General Practitioners also make positive and valuable suggestions, and these are recommended for further reading.

Role of the Primary Health Care Team

Primary health care is a much broader concept than the medical and nursing care provided by general practitioners and nurses. The main principles underlying the Declaration of Alma Ata in 1978 and endorsed by the World Health Assembly in May 1979 are that primary health care should:

- be built on the principle of community participation
- be staffed by a multidisciplinary team
- serve as first point of contact to the national health system
- be supported by an effective referral system
- prevent disease, promote health, treat illness, care and rehabilitate
- maintain a continuity of relationship with every member of the population it serves
- reach out into all homes and workplaces systematically to identify those at highest risk
- help people to assume greater responsibility for their own health.

The term 'Primary Health Care Team' describes all those working in association with general practitioners, nurses and health visitors from health centres or other premises and includes secretaries, receptionists and lay participants. Membership is flexible and could at any time include dietitians, psychologists, health education officers and others. Important aspects of the Team's role are:

- raising people's awareness of health and the importance of lifestyle
- identifying and monitoring people at special risk
- taking a responsible attitude towards the community regarding the control of risks and treatment of related disease.

A shortage of relevant skills and resources is an important constraint if the Primary Health Care Team is to respond energetically to prevention. Appropriate training is needed together with the support of staff trained in epidemiology, and in the collecting and storing of information. Key members such as health visitors are in short supply, and proposals to capitalise on their skills and role will mean urgent attention to staffing levels. Marshalling the available skills is further complicated by different management arrangements for different Team members. Nurses and health visitors are responsible to the District Health Authority while general practitioners are independent contractors with Family Practitioner Committees.

Members of the Primary Health Care Team in the United Kingdom have distinct professional identities, with very different methods of recruitment, training and certification. The creation of a new type of member may therefore be resisted by sectors of some professions. For example, a general practitioner may wish to appoint someone with special experience and skills as a 'prevention practice nurse'. Because the Primary Health Care Team is a response to the community's health needs and not there of its own right, such developments should not be discouraged if they are required.

It is important to emphasise that whilst the prevention of coronary heart disease is a major priority for the Team, it should not be seen in isolation to other activities of health promotion and disease prevention. Action directed at the prevention and control of smoking, hypertension and obesity, and the promotion of healthy nutrition and exercise is also likely to have major impacts on other areas of health care, for example, the prevention of stroke, cancer, respiratory and dental disease.

Motivating the Primary Health Care Team

If the prevention of coronary heart disease is to become a major priority for the work of Primary Health Care Teams, a major realignment of thought and practice will be required amongst many of them. Changes in the philosophy, attitude and behaviour of Team members, could be initiated in a variety of ways. Important examples are as follows:

1. Involvement in District Planning

Active participation of Team members in the planning of District prevention policies is highly motivating and can be reinforced by suitable articles in health journals. (See also Chapter Four.)

2. Organisation of Educational Initiatives

Local seminars could be organised on prevention in which all members of the 'extended' Team are invited to take part. The prevention initiatives of the Royal College of General Practitioners, emphasised and rein-forced by the local College Faculties and their Clinical Tutors, could play an influential part in this process. Practice 'audits' of preventive practice could also be of benefit.

3. Production of a Practice Report

This could be done on an annual basis and should include the work of the whole of the Team. The form of the report should be decided in consultation with all those working in the Team and those in the District Health Authority with responsibility for preventive services. The advice of health education officers, dietitians and health visitors could add substantially to the report's value.

4. Appointment of an Information Officer

A person with expertise in the extraction and use of information could be appointed by the general practice itself or could be seconded to the Team by the District Health Authority. Community physicians could offer their skills and resources particularly in the development of appro-priate epidemiology (health status monitoring etc).

5. Use of a Health Promotion 'Facilitator' and Liaison Person

A facilitator could be very valuable in encouraging and helping the practice to provide a more effective preventive service. This could be a person provided by the District Health Authority or someone appointed by the practice or a group of practices. The concept of a Primary Health Care Team liaison person to stimulate, support and co-ordinate activities is also referred to in Chapters Four and Six.

6. Development of General Practitioners with a Special Interest

The encouragement of general practitioners to develop special interests and expertise in the field of prevention and health promotion could also be particularly helpful. These doctors, perhaps called 'Primary Community Physicians', could liaise closely with the District Medical Officer and could play an integral part in developing the District's preventive and information services. Viewing the practice 'list' as a population and adopting a community approach, they could be an effective means of providing preventive services and stimulating change within the community on a wide number of fronts.

7. Involvement of Consumer or Lay Groups

Expressions of community needs and concerns by Consumer (patient) groups and associations can be a powerful force in stimulating change. Groups can be particularly useful in developing health education strategies by bridging the gap between the 'professionals' and the local population, and can also help monitor programmes. Their development could be encouraged and supported. The need for combined lay and professional inputs at local level to form neighbourhood groups for health promotion has already been discussed in Chapter Four.

Recommendations

The following proposals are made to support and enhance the preventive activities of the Primary Health Care Team. In view of the very different circumstances pertaining to individual members, the recommendations should be regarded and used as 'Guidelines of Good Practice' rather than definitive instructions.

1. Planning for Health Promotion

(i)   Representatives from Primary Health Care Teams, the community, and Community Health Councils should take an active and early part in the planning and implementation of District policies and strategies for health promotion, particularly the prevention of coronary heart disease. The appointment of a Primary Care Team liaison person within the District to stimulate, support and co-ordinate activities is essential. (See also Chapters Four and Six.)

(ii) Improvements in the management and organisation of general practice should be given much greater emphasis, as this is crucial to the provision of an effective preventive service. General practitioners and practice managers should be encouraged to increase their expertise in these areas. Reception and secretarial services in the practice should be made available to all the Team professionals, and any extra workload created should be spread among all of them.

(iii) Manpower resources should be used more efficiently and less rigidly. Team members employed by the District Health Authority should as far as possible be allowed to establish long-term working relationships with colleagues, clients and patients. Community physicians should actively co-operate with Teams and share their resources and skills.

(iv) Primary health care premises should be seen as a community resource for health (i.e. the provision of information, guidance and services for the promotion of health). In addition to consultation rooms, clinical facilities and waiting areas etc, facilities need to be provided for community meetings, group counselling sessions and keep-fit classes, etc. A medium-sized meeting room, and changing and showering facilities would therefore be valuable. Planners should recognise these requirements when building Health Centres or their equivalent.

(v)   Customer groups commonly known as 'patient participation groups' serving a general practice or health centre should be encouraged and developed. Neighbourhood groups for health promotion incorporating both lay and professional inputs, should be established (see Chapter Four).

2. Primary Health Care Team Members

(i)   Health visitors are vital for the successful implementation of preventive policies. They should maintain a strong link with the District Health Education Unit. Their work should be included in a practice annual report which they should help compile. However, if health visitors are to be expected to fulfil their potential role in prevention, health education and health promotion, then their numbers must be considerably increased. A goal of one health visitor to 2,000 total population is therefore proposed.

(ii)   Midwives and nurses in the Primary Health Care Team are also in an ideal position to be health educators as the prevention of coronary disease needs to be on a broad front — directed as much to the family as to the individual. They need additional training in counselling and health education.

(iii)   The skills offered by community or hospital-based dietitians should be used more widely by the Team. Their guidance should be sought in establishing policy and advice on the dietary aspects of coronary heart disease prevention and weight reduction. A close relationship often exists between dietitians and health education officers, and this is a convenient way in which contact can be established.

(iv)   The general practitioner is seen by many as an authoritative and effective means by which health risk advice can be conveyed to people. Although an increasing number are developing a preventive role, the level and form of activity could be improved. The development of counselling and communication skills is important, and general practitioners should be encouraged to be trained in these fields.

3. Developing Links with the District Health Education Unit

(i)   A close working relationship should be built between health education officers and members of Primary Health Care Teams. Health visitors have an important part to play here.

(ii) Health education officers should be included in the planning of health education and health promotion strategies within primary health care. They have skills and resources which would be of enormous benefit to the Team.

(iii) One of the main difficulties in promoting these types of link is the lack of channels of communication and the barriers which frequently arise between professional disciplines. The District Health Authority could help by introducing general practitioners into the early stages of health education and health promotion planning as recommended earlier and in Chapter Four.

(iv) Health education officers should be invited to organise seminars and small group work on health promotion for members of Teams. As well as improving knowledge and skills, such activities should remove barriers and improve communication between health workers. (See also Chapter Six.)

4. Detecting and Managing People at High Risk

(i) An assessment of each individual's risk of coronary heart disease should be made by the general practitioner and this should be recorded in the person's records. At-risk registers should be kept and used and follow-up mechanisms should be developed. The most relevant factors to include, apart from age and sex, are family history, occupation/social class, smoking history, weight, blood pressure and (if available) serum cholesterol. Cumulative risks accrue from the use of oral contraceptives, and the presence of diabetic states and glucose intolerance. It is particularly important to take note of all these factors in the first degree relatives of patients with coronary heart disease occurring under the age of 55 years.

(ii) Regular information about smoking habits should be recorded for all people from an early age. A major effort should be made to increase the public's awareness of the risks of smoking. Support and help for those wishing to stop smoking should be offered (including where appropriate referral to smoking cessation groups and clinics). Anti-smoking activities should be an integral part of a broader approach within the District (see Chapter Four). An information system is necessary to gather data from various sources including primary care about the smoking habits of the individual and the community.

(iii) Height and weight measurements to detect those with excess
       weight should be made whenever possible. Dietary changes can be
       made and healthy eating habits established much more easily at a
       younger age, and so the earlier the detection the better. People
       should be encouraged to weigh themselves regularly so that they
       themselves can aim to achieve optimal weight for height. When
       indicated appropriate dietary advice should be offered during
       consultations. Dietitians should where possible be available for
       individual consultations. Support groups to help weight loss should
       be developed. The needs of men should not be overlooked.
       Information about weight control groups should be available at
       health centres and practices.

(iv)   The risk of coronary heart disease is greater when blood choles-
       terol is high (and related lipoproteins are abnormal), especially
       where there is familial hyper-cholesterolaemia. The Team should
       therefore try to identify hyper-cholesterolaemic individuals by
       screening families with premature vascular disease. Blood lipids
       should be measured in first degree relatives of patients who
       develop coronary heart disease under 55 years and particularly
       under 50. Appropriate dietary or other intervention can then be
       initiated. Attention to other risk factors is also particularly
       important in these individuals.

(v)   Where possible exercise habits should be discussed and recorded.
       The development of regular and suitable exercise should be
       advised where appropriate. Information about the existence and
       place of various forms of exercise groups, and about sports and
       exercise facilities in the locality, should be prominently displayed
       in health centres and practices. When new Team premises are being
       planned some effort should be made to relate these to sports and
       community centres.

(vi)   Although more research is required into the part that stress might
       play in ill health, there is much that could be done to encourage
       people to develop methods to respond to stress. Opportunities
       should be taken during consultations to talk about the need for
       adequate relaxation, and information about how this can be
       achieved should be made available.

(vii) As trends in blood pressure are important, the Team should be
       encouraged to take measurements during adult life. These could
       start at school-leaving age. Blood pressure recordings should be
       made approximately every five years unless more frequent
       recordings are necessary as part of the management of raised
       blood pressure. Facilities for taking and recording blood pressure

should be easily accessible and in certain situations self-recording by patients may be feasible.

Blood pressure which is moderately raised does not necessarily require treatment by drugs, which can cause problems. It may well be quite adequate to manage less severe hypertension by modifying lifestyle, e.g. by reducing weight, salt consumption and alcohol intake, and by increasing exercise. Measuring blood pressure also offers an opportunity for counselling and discussion of other risk factors for coronary heart disease.

Measurements of blood pressure should always be recorded. Any community-based blood pressure screening programme should be designed so that the results of individual patients can be made available to the general practitioner concerned.

The provision of services for blood pressure recording, whether by the Team or by the Community Health Service, should be closely monitored. Age and sex related information concerning the prevalence of hypertension in the community should be made available to the Primary Health Care Teams and the District Health Authority.

(viii) All those working in primary health care should be aware of the possibilities of alcohol misuse and should discuss drinking habits during consultations. Major efforts should be made to raise the public's awareness of what constitutes safe drinking. Priority should be given to identifying those at greatest risk. Sustained help should be offered to those with an alcohol problem, and a close relationship should be established between the Team and the relevant helping agencies.

5. Improving Records and Information Systems

(i) More emphasis should be put on using the data accumulated by Primary Health Care Teams. Complete and clear health records of the individual are crucial for preventive activity. Records should include information obtained by *all* members of the Team.

(ii) Standard A4 size record folders should be adopted. These would improve the keeping of records and their use, for example in the building up of 'at risk' and morbidity registers, and the transfer of information to a computer base.

(iii) The establishment of a data base and the retrieval of information within primary health care is important for both planning and monitoring. Although preventive services can be provided in the

absence of 'age/sex' and 'at risk' registers, these approaches allow
the initiation, monitoring and follow-up of specific preventive
activities, and should therefore be developed. A practice report
should be published regularly, preferably annually. This should be
the responsibility of a skilled member of the Team; either a
general practitioner, a person appointed under the reimbursed
ancillary staff scheme, or someone shared with the District Health
Authority.

(iv) The feed-back of health status information to both health professionals and the community they serve can act as an important
reinforcement to health education messages. This task should be
a District Health Authority responsibility. A District health profile about coronary heart disease should include wherever possible
mortality and morbidity rates, the prevalence of risk factors, the
level of provision of services, and the uptake of screening facilities.

6. Developing Professional Education and Training

(i) Universities and colleges responsible for teaching health professionals should combine the principles of health promotion and
disease prevention into all their curricula. This extension should
be reflected in all relevant professional examinations.

However, the undergraduate and postgraduate teaching of those
involved in prevention will be difficult in the near future. This is
because there are so few teachers in medical, dental and nursing
schools with the necessary experience, approach and skills. The
Departments of General Practice and Community Medicine within universities should therefore play a major role in developing
necessary teaching skills. The Royal Colleges should also consider developing national policies for better training in prevention.

(ii) Vocational training for general practitioners should include
clinical epidemiology appropriate to primary care, the theory
and practice of prevention, health education and the promotion
of health. This could well be undertaken in conjunction with
other disciplines who are concerned with primary health care.

(iii) In-service training in the methods of prevention and health promotion, and in counselling and communication techniques,
should be developed for all primary care health professionals. It
is particularly important that all those working in primary health
care should be able to work together as a team.

(iv) One criterion for the appointment of general practitioner trainers should be that they have the facilities for developing and undertaking preventive activities in their practices.

(v) A Manual of Prevention and Health Promotion should be produced for Primary Health Care Teams. This should address itself to the special needs of primary health care workers and to the development of an appropriate epidemiological approach to health promotion and disease prevention. This would not only be of great practical use but would also be an important motivating force. The Royal College of General Practitioners and the Health Visitors' Association, together with the Department of Health should commission such an initiative.

7. Research

(i) There is a rapidly increasing need for co-ordinated research into methods of prevention and the means of implementing preventive strategies. The results of such studies should be disseminated widely to all in primary health care work.

(ii) Primary health care professionals should also participate in research. Such work can be highly motivating, as shown by the continuing effects of the Medical Research Council's Mild to Moderate Hypertension Trial.

Chapter Six
ACTION THROUGH HEALTH EDUCATION

Health education is an integral part of all activities to prevent coronary heart disease – at national, Regional, District and Primary Care Team levels. It includes any activity which promotes health-related learning and some relatively permanent change in health action of individuals, groups and institutions. Health education may produce changes in understanding, ways of thinking, belief and attitude, and may facilitate the acquisition of skills. Importantly, it may help generate changes in individual behaviour and life style, and improvements in the wider socio-economic environment that influence health.

Health education's role in prevention must be closely integrated with other actions designed to reduce both individual and population levels of risk. The most effective health education may come from strategies which both help individuals and encourage social change and community action. This chapter briefly considers four major approaches to health education and the need for long and short term outcomes. It then discusses organisational aspects and the role of key agencies. Finally recommendations are made which are practically orientated to achieve action in the short term.

Choice of Health Education Approaches

Within the various schools of thought on health education that are now emerging, there seem to be four major categories of approach. The Health Education Council is currently developing practical applications of these. Each approach has its own advantages and disadvantages which are summarised as follows:

- **Health Risk Advice**

  Seeks to use medical/scientific information and advice to achieve behaviour changes conducive to health in individuals. This is the most widely used approach and has been dominant for a long time. The over-reliance on this so-called 'medical model' has been questioned both because of doubts over its effectiveness in some areas of activity and its emphasis on 'expert' views imposed upon vulnerable individuals.

- **Personal self-empowerment**

  Seeks to build self-esteem and increase the learner's social and life skills. Unlike the 'medical' model, it focuses on learning processes which can assist the individual to make healthy choices. The approach is non-authoritarian and is indirect in its effect on health. These attributes, plus the long period before results would be expected to show, make evaluation difficult.

- **Public Agenda-setting**

  Seeks to increase awareness amongst the public, professionals and policy makers of the size and nature of health problems. It encourages debate on the need for and means of beneficial change, taking into account individual lifestyle, health service provision and the socio-economic environment. Like the health risk advice approach it has a potential disadvantage of being too expert-dominated. Because the approach operates within many complex processes of social change, it is difficult to evaluate.

- **Community Action Development**

  Seeks to encourage and support local and neighbourhood groups to take health promoting actions they themselves have identified as being important. The role of the educator here may be chiefly in offering resources and help so that communities may develop their full potential in winning health for themselves.

  It is beyond the scope of this report to enter into a theoretical discussion of the various health education approaches. There is a large literature which was usefully reviewed for the conference by Alan Beattie (1983).

The choice of health education approaches to use in the prevention of coronary heart disease depends on the particular educational objectives; the setting; the skills, resources and support available to health educators; and the timescale. Self-empowerment and community action approaches will probably be more effective in the long term in reducing coronary heart disease. For instance, 'Lifeskills Teaching' has been developed in many school curricula and is designed to help people to resist social pressures to smoke. Other, more general teaching, designed to enhance self-esteem could be expected to improve the likelihood of people responding to invitations to 'look after themselves' and avoid a variety of health risks including those associated with coronary heart disease.

However, given the importance of coronary heart disease in the UK, it is essential to consider health education actions which can be expected to bring results in the short term as well as the long term. The health risk advice and public agenda-setting approaches thus also have a place. The added advantage of combining all four approaches, is that a number of different health education agencies and settings can contribute to prevention. For example, a school is in a better position to teach life-skills than a Primary Health Care Team. On the other hand, a general practitioner may be ideally suited to provide authoritative advice on the need to stop smoking to a high-risk patient, and give the necessary support. Nevertheless there are dangers in over-emphasising the negative aspects of particular lifestyles. A more general approach, which focuses on the positive benefits of exercise, healthy eating and stress management, has the attraction of being designed primarily to make people feel better while incidentally reducing the risks of coronary heart disease.

The prevention of coronary heart disease thus requires a combination of the four major approaches, which should be seen as complementary. All health educators should be fully aware of these approaches, their advantages and disadvantages and their most appropriate uses. All agencies (e.g. Health Education Units, Primary Care Teams, schools, adult education, the media, etc) should know what particular contributions they can make in a global health education strategy.

Organisational Aspects

A major initiative organised as a single campaign across the nation is unlikely to be the most appropriate strategy. The lessons from the successful Stanford and North Karelia programmes suggest that District and Regional strategies are likely to be the most effective. Experimental programmes — such as that envisaged in Wales by the Health Education Council — are welcomed. The development of locally based programmes has already been emphasised in Chapter Four and will therefore only be discussed briefly here.

1. A District Strategy

A wide variety of organisations and groups are concerned with health education activities at a District level, and these need to be harnessed for the prevention of coronary heart disease by the District Health Authority. The nature, extent and sophistication of the activities will vary considerably. There are differences between the kind of health education that can be offered at schools and health centres, as well as differences in the degree of involvement and commitment amongst the professionals concerned.

Three main principles emerge from these observations:

   (i) Each agency should be expected to make an educational contribution consistent with its expertise and the kind of contact it has with the public.

(ii) Those agencies not fulfilling their potential health education function should be encouraged to do so.

(iii) The activities of all agencies should be identified and co-ordinated.

An integrated, co-ordinated and effective programme of health education at District level is essential.

2. Regional Strategy

Although the main focus of activity will be within Districts, Regional support will be necessary. The structure and services required have already been outlined in Chapter Four. Of particular benefit to health education initiatives will be a strengthened information base; co-ordinated press, public relations and general media support; and research facilities. Studies of the major coronary heart disease prevention programmes, such as the Stanford and North Karelia projects, have shown that even a regional media-based programme without a receptive local infrastructure is unlikely to have a significant impact.

The appointment of an appropriately trained health professional (Regional Health Promotion Officer) to co-ordinate and extend activities at Regional level is seen as essential.

3. National Support

In several countries non-governmental national organisations dedicated to the prevention of coronary heart disease have played a crucial role in raising public awareness in the community. This activity has ultimately led to the involvement of statutory health and education services in specific coronary heart disease prevention programmes. Support at national level from organisations such as these could be particularly helpful to health educators.

The government-funded Health Education Council will continue to have an important role at national level in co-ordination, information provision and support with mass media work, resource and curricula development, and training. In addition to its existing coronary heart disease prevention programmes, many other Council projects are already concerned with heart disease risk factors. The Council could usefully extend all of these activities, and especially enhance its role as a national clearing house for resources for use by the various agencies. The Council will need to be more sensitive to local needs, and this will require some regionalisation of activities as already mentioned in Chapter Four. The Council's plans for an experimental programme in Sales should be particularly helpful in providing new information on the most effective and efficient ways of delivering health education.

Role of Key Agencies

A range of organisations and groups are already concerned directly or indirectly in health education which could reduce the risk of heart disease. Five of the most important (the school, adult and community education, primary care, the workplace and the mass media) are considered in this section, with the aim of highlighting opportunities for development. If they do not already exist, links will need to be forged with the groups and the District Heart Disease Prevention Team and its partner Health Education Service.

1. The School

The school is a major focal point for health education, but a specific heart disease prevention programme in schools would probably be inappropriate. However, it is important to recognise that existing general education and more specific health education programmes already contribute to the prevention of coronary heart disease. Much can be done within existing curricula to meet this goal. Biology, home economics and physical education already play a part. Personal and social education such as 'Lifeskills Teaching' can make an important contribution, for instance, by teaching social skills and enhancing self-esteem. Both processes can help young people resist social pressures to take health risks and, less obviously, provide the conviction and skills necessary to take communal action to improve health. More specifically, a large number of schools currently offer one or more of the existing school-based health education projects. Some consider coronary heart disease as a specific issue and all focus on major risk factors. These include the '5–13', '13–18', 'Slow Learners', 'My Body', 'Active Tutorial Work Development', 'Lifeskills and Health Education', and 'Smoking Education for Teenagers' projects sponsored and developed by the Health Education Council. It is important that teachers appreciate the rationale behind these projects as regards education for personal development, education for ecological and political understanding, and education for community service.

Thus the key tasks for the District Health Education Service and Local Education Authority Advisory Service, will be to co-ordinate existing activities and extend them where appropriate. No opportunities should be lost to involve all parts of the school community, including Parent/Teacher Associations and also the school health service which, as yet, has no clear role in supporting health education.

2. Adult and Community Education

Very diverse centres provide adult and community education, including formal adult education evening classes, and less formal community-based programmes. The Health Education Council's 'Look After Yourself' adult education programme, focusing on coronary risk factors, is nationwide and continues to develop. The key task is again to co-ordinate and extend activities. There will be a need to identify relevant existing courses, and tutors or leaders who can be used in health education. Tutors will need to understand the underlying concepts of this form of health education. These comprise helping adults to learn how to safeguard their own health and the health of the community. This can be achieved by improving their personal and social skills, by widening their understanding of what is needed for a healthy environment, and by directing them outwards into community networks and lines of self-help action.

3. Primary Health Care

The scope for health education in primary health care is becoming widely acknowledged. Numerous opportunities exist in the day-to-day contacts of the Primary Health Care Team with the public. However, because consultation time is limited, the general practitioner and other members of the Team need to make maximum use of these opportunities. This calls for improved communication skills coupled with effective team work. For example, the obese individual who is given clear and specific dietary advice, or an invitation to join a practice-based weight reduction group, is more likely to take action than someone offered vague advice "to try to lose a bit of weight". Such activities can be further supported by a well-organised practice information system which highlights patients and families at risk (e.g. those smoking, obese, or with a raised blood pressure), and which enables longer term monitoring and evaluation of preventive activities. Chapter Five has already discussed these developments.

4. The Workplace

Health education in the workplace poses special problems of access, time and facilities. Health educators will need to present their case convincingly to both management and the workforce.

Management may be persuaded by evidence from the USA that health education initiatives and improved occupational health care can result in greater productivity, less paid sickness absence and, in most cases, greater corporate identity. For the workforce, a strengthened occupational health service and improved working conditions can be viewed as important fringe benefits. Occupational health staff can be the key contacts but they are found generally only in larger companies. In smaller firms, where there are no permanent occupational health staff other strategies need to be employed, such as through a direct approach to management or personnel departments. Environmental Health Officers could be useful allies in gaining access to the workplace. Heart Disease Prevention Teams should attempt to work closely with the local Environmental Health Department.

5. Mass Media

Health educators will need to consider the purposeful use of the mass media as one part of a planned programme of health education. (See also Chapter Seven.) The use of the media, particularly advertising, has been de-emphasised recently in the UK because of rather disappointing results from often over-ambitious and unco-ordinated national campaigns. Lessons from overseas, however, show that careful and co-ordinated use of the media has an important role in promoting public awareness and interest in the community (agenda-setting). They can be used to achieve specific health objectives if a supportive local infrastructure exists (e.g. the Health Education Council 'Superman' campaign). Districts should take every opportunity to use the media in local initiatives. Press and public relations officers within the National Health Service, who are usually based at Regional level, can offer much advice and support. In view of the large media overlaps between Districts, a budget for mass media campaigns needs to be available at Regional level. However, it should be stressed that if this resource is to be used successfully, there must be a receptive local infrastructure to capitalise on any initiatives. (See also Chapter Four.)

Recommendations

1. Strategy

(i) Health education approaches for the prevention of coronary heart disease should include health risk advice, personal self-empowerment, public agenda-setting and community action development. Such a combination would be expected to achieve short term as well as longer lasting change.

(ii) All health and educational agencies and professionals should contribute to health education programmes for the prevention of coronary heart disease.

These include teachers, general practitioners, health visitors, community nurses, hospital medical and nursing staff, dietitians, physiotherapists and health education officers. They should be aware of their particular responsibilities and contributions, and the range of health education approaches available. Training both pre- and post-qualification should be increased considerably. Professional bodies as well as health and education authorities should consider as a matter of urgency their responsibilities for ensuring that professionals are appropriately trained.

In Districts where there is no specialist health education presence, urgent attention and priority should be given to establishing and developing one. The District Health Education Service and its staff will frequently form the cornerstone of many of the activities recommended and it must be viewed as an essential component of any District Health Authority.

The appointment of a health education officer to work in the field of community action (development) is essential as has been recommended in Chapter Four.

(iii) A multidisciplinary steering group for health education should be established as a sub-group of the District Heart Disease Prevention Team. The key task will be to co-ordinate and extend activities within the wide range of opportunities that exist at local level. The group should be flexible in its approach and free from bureaucratic constraints. It should not consist of 'routinely' appointed *ex-officio* members of existing authorities but rather should include the best local expertise. It will need to work in close co-operation with the District Health Education Unit which should be represented on the group.

(iv) As the District Heart Disease Prevention Team is likely to be more of an advisory or steering group for local initiatives, it should have sufficient funding to appoint co-ordinators – possibly on a seconded basis – and cover expenses. These co-ordinators would include the additional health education officer (community development) and primary care co-ordinator suggested in Chapter Four. However, there may also be a need to involve workers from outside the NHS – for example, a community exercise co-ordinator seconded from a local authority. It must be stressed that such people can only be considered as catalysts for existing resources and manpower.

(v) Support from Regional Health Authorities and the Health Education Council should be available, particularly for the provision of resources and support materials, the production and co-ordination of mass media initiatives, and assistance with training, research and monitoring.

2. Schools

(i)   The Health Education Council should continue investment in the dissemination of the current school health education projects. This would not only widen the use of existing materials, but, as part of a programme of in-service education for teachers, it could also highlight specific coronary heart disease issues within the school context.

(ii) As part of this process, more schools should appoint a health education co-ordinator from within their own staff. (Over 50 per cent of secondary schools currently have co-ordinators.) The role of such a teacher should be to review and co-ordinate existing activity and, in addition, to examine wider school policies and practices related to health, such as the school shop, school meals, staff smoking etc.

(iii) Although schools will be mainly concerned with more general approaches to health education, specific learning resources on the prevention of coronary heart disease could be useful. The Health Education Council should develop and publish such a teaching package, either drawing substantially on existing materials or through an extension of existing projects.

3. Adult and Community Education

(i)   An adult education co-ordinator should be identified within each District. Working closely with local health education officers such a person could be responsible for co-ordinating existing activity in adult and community education as well as acting as a catalyst for new initiatives specific to the prevention of coronary heart disease.

(ii) The Health Education Council's 'Look After Yourself' (LAY) adult education project should be further extended and developed, particularly in marketing the course to the general public. This will mean more extensive client advertising than previously, as well as providing training for additional LAY tutors. To aid recruitment further, the courses and training need to be more flexible both in terms of content and accessibility (i.e. not exclusively through 'Adult Education Classes').

4. Primary Health Care

(i)   Closer links should be established between the District Health

Education Unit and the local postgraduate centres, possibly through the Primary Health Care Team liaison person. (See also Chapters Four and Five.) A programme of meetings should be arranged concerning such key issues as improving communication and team-skills, and establishing practice information systems.

(ii) The resources available to general practitioners and health visitors for health risk advice should be extended and developed. These might include a re-launch of the Health Education Council's 'Give Up Smoking' pack and the development and publication of sensible exercise and healthy eating pamphlets.

5. The Workplace

(i) The Health Education Council should produce an in-service training package for occupational health staff. This should concern general health education as well as prevention of coronary heart disease. Content should include highlighting opportunities for health education, improving personal skills and suggesting initiatives.

(ii) The Health Education Council should consider producing specific mass media materials for use in the workplace as such materials are presently lacking. The Open University adoption of 'health choices' and 'Look After Yourself' materials for use in industry could be explored.

6. The Media

(i) The media should be used to the full in both opportunistic ways, as well as part of a planned sequence of activities. Regional budgets will be required (see Chapter Four). District Heart Disease Prevention Teams should encourage the local media to take up prepared programmes (e.g. a Health Education Council local radio package) or to design and produce locally-based programmes.

(ii) A number of key 'spokesmen' should be identified by the Heart Disease Prevention Team and be given additional training in the use of the media (specifically radio and television interview techniques). This will allow for better and more controlled opportunistic use of the local media.

(iii) District Heart Disease Prevention Teams should consider the more specific use of the media for certain issues (e.g. helping smokers to give up). Full consideration will need to be given to the provision of adequate support services to meet the public demand, which will be created by the use of the media in this way. (See also Chapter Seven.)

7. Smoking Prevention

(i) Schools should adopt a smoking prevention policy, perhaps based on the forthcoming survey and guidelines from the Health Education Council. As part of a wider review of the 'health' curriculum, schools should consider using the Council's 'Smoking Education for Teenagers' project.

(ii) The Health Education Council together with other research bodies should commission research into specific strategies for helping older teenagers to give up smoking.

(iii) More resources should be made available to locally-based groups that encourage community action to promote non-smoking (e.g. ASH, GASP). The Heart Disease Prevention Team should also consider the provision of smoking cessation facilities in the community and the possibility of establishing a network of stop-smoking self-help groups.

(iv) Updated lists of smoking cessation facilities should be made available to the Primary Health Care Teams. Some general practitioners or health visitors might also consider setting up practice-based smoking cessation groups.

(v) Heart Disease Prevention Teams should urge local firms to implement fair smoking policies, with adequate facilities for non-smokers. There may be scope for the production of a 'Give Up Smoking at Work' kit based on the general practice 'Give Up Smoking' model. Larger firms might also consider the feasibility of work-based smoking cessation groups.

8. Healthy Nutrition Promotion

(i) A simplified version of the NACNE report on dietary guidelines should be produced for schools. This could be used as the basis for teaching healthy nutrition as well as offering specific guidance on the choice of nutritionally-sound school meals.

(ii) A District food and health policy should be developed and implemented throughout the community. This should provide firm guidelines for community action. Heart Disease Prevention Teams should also consider the feasibility of local community nutrition schemes.

(iii) Heart Disease Prevention Teams should ensure that diet plans and leaflets are available for use by Primary Health Care Teams. They should also provide updated lists of reputable weight reduction groups. General practitioners and health visitors should also consider setting up their own practice-based weight reduction groups.

(iv) Firms should be urged to implement healthy eating policies in canteens (possibly with subsidised 'healthy' foods). All occupational health departments should have weighing machinery for use by the workforce and some may consider the provision of work-based weight reduction groups.

9. Exercise Promotion

(i) Schools should adopt the Physical Education Association guidelines (1979) as school policy. These emphasise the principle of sport for all and stress the important role of schools in equipping young people with the basic skills necessary to take part in a wide range of physical activities.

(ii) The Heart Disease Prevention Team should produce, in collaboration with local authorities and sports councils, information on facilities and programmes of exercise suitable for a wide range of ages and abilities. This information should be widely accessible in public places, health centres, etc, and should also be presented personally to all health visitors and general practitioners in the District. Teams should also consider establishing a small exercise sponsorship fund to foster innovative community exercise events and programmes.

(iii) Firms should be urged to provide facilities so that staff are able to exercise before and after work and during lunch periods. These might include the provision of some basic equipment and showers. Occupational health staff might also be able to supervise a simple fitness-testing scheme (e.g. Harvard Fitness Step Test) and provide individual guidance to employees on ways to improve physical fitness.

(iv) At national level the Health Education Council should join forces with the Sports Council in the promotion of sensible exercise, particularly amongst low activity groups. Common strategies should be agreed, and some pooling of resources could be helpful.

Chapter Seven
ACTION THROUGH THE MASS MEDIA

Expectations of change as a result of the use of the media must be realistic. The media inform, and they can change attitudes, especially in the short term, but they will not usually affect behaviour except when supported by other influences such as personal education and development, provision of services, legislation, taxation, and community action.

'The media' as referred to in this chapter include television, radio, newspapers, magazines, books and leaflets, and the use of advertising and marketing techniques. The media can be further divided into local, regional and national, according to target audiences. The term 'media professionals' refers to all media workers with editorial responsibility.

Health promotion through the media needs to emphasise positive not negative messages. For example, rather than recommending people to eat less fat, sugar and salt and more fibre, it would be better to state this advice positively by emphasising the advantages of an increase in consumption of fresh fruit and vegetables, wholemeal and other bread, and cereals generally.

The promotion of 'healthy living' is likely to be more attractive to the public than the prevention of specific diseases, about which public knowledge is limited. There is advantage then in developing general health programmes within which specific diseases such as coronary heart disease can be discussed. The observation of lifestyle and environmental changes associated with alterations in incidence of these diseases in many industrial countries is impressive and reinforces the message for action.

Many processes within the media are relatively difficult to describe clearly. This chapter, therefore, concentrates on those media issues for which firm, feasible and positive recommendations can be presented.

Representation of Health Issues in the Media

An important step in using the media to assist in the prevention of coronary heart disease, is to shift the balance of content towards health promotion. It is feasible to heighten the profile of health promotion in news coverage but this requires specific effort from health promoters. News coverage is event-related but it should be appreciated that a great deal of news can be, and is, 'manufactured'.

Much of health coverage is through 'medical correspondents' and the technology and science of medicine tend to dominate — for example, transplants, body scanners, and drug scares. This emphasises disease and treatment, and the promotion of health or disease-avoidance has a low priority. The agenda of the media need to be shifted from promoting 'medicine' to promoting 'health'.

Incorrect or inaccurate information in stories can be more harmful than no coverage. Fear of such 'mis-reporting' deters many health workers from using the media fully. Nevertheless many opportunities are lost for coverage which could be overcome if health professionals were better trained in the use of the media. Table II outlines some provisional 'Handy Hints for Health Professionals' when giving interviews to the media.

TABLE II. Handy Hints for Health Promoters

1. Where possible, provide printed material for a talk or conference, e.g. make available copies of your speech. This makes it easier for the media to understand your points and harder to misquote you.

2. Try to meet the journalist or producer you are dealing with in person, rather than talking exclusively over the phone.

3. Try to discover the general purpose of the message of the programme or article being considered. Decide how your views are likely to fit in. Are you going to be presented as the single exponent of one cause, as a crank, as the 'baddie' in the journalist's or producer's scenario?

4. Establish the basis of the discussion right at the start, i.e. whether it is 'off the record' or for quotation. Some journalists are happy to talk at length 'off the record' and then work out a summary of what is acceptable to both sides for quotation.

5. Be as straightforward and honest as possible. If a journalist feels that you are trying to hide something, misunderstandings may result.

6. Cultivate certain individuals in the media. If a journalist feels he may get another story from you, he is likely to take particular trouble to get the story right.

It is wrong to assume that media professionals, specialist or non-specialist, have all the right contacts, or up-to-date knowledge of the particular field, or access to the latest and appropriate reference material. They endeavour to ascertain the facts but they are often working to deadlines which do not allow sufficient time to develop expertise. Many also work on their own. Health promoters should accept their responsibility to fill these gaps by providing the necessary professional input in a way which is relevant to the user.

There is substantial evidence that the media, especially television drama, have a marked influence on the choices people make about their habits and lifestyle. However, like some doctors, many media professionals do not feel it is their responsibility to influence in a positive way attitudes and behaviour. This view needs to be changed. For example, many small incidental aspects of drama production – location, smoking and drinking behaviour, attitudes to foods, etc – could be modified easily if the media professionals saw the possible health advantages. The same incidentals could be chosen to reinforce health promotion programmes rather than being neutral or in conflict (e.g. Superman does not smoke).

Planned Use of the Media

In addition to opportunistic coverage of health issues, there can be planned and purposeful use of the media. This can be initiated either by the media professional or by a health professional (individual, group or organisation). In many cases, the idea for a programme or articles will come from an individual producer or journalist, who might then enlist the help and advice of outside people and bodies. Interested groups or individual health professionals can suggest a topic or try to influence the approach to a subject. But form and content will remain very much in the editorial control of the producer or writer. It is unrealistic for outside groups to expect to have more than a marginal influence on this process.

However, an increasing number of media projects involve more elaborate and sophisticated collaboration with non-media groups. These are occasionally initiated by outside groups who hope to involve press or broadcasters in a larger project, incorporating various community activities. The success of such partnerships depends on a joint agreement about the desirability and feasibility of the project, and on the availability of resources.

Health and media professionals could help each other by achieving a better understanding of each other's role and needs. As good journalism requires good contacts, appropriate directories could be prepared. The Health Education Council could provide a more comprehensive information service so that the media can easily contact the appropriate agency or person.

All Regional Health Authorities have public relations officers although only a minority of Districts have such posts. There is great variation between Regions in the emphasis given to health promotion by the Authority and hence in the role of the public relations officers. Most Regions act reactively to the media and the scope for initiating work with the media could be examined. The example of energetic out-reach for health promotion by the press and public relations departments of Wessex and West Midlands Regional Health Authorities could be replicated in other Regions. Paid advertising in the UK has been used to publicise health events and meetings, to raise public awareness, and to seek specific behavioural changes. The latter objective has often failed as a result of insufficient back-up, poor market research and lack of community-based supporting programmes. The concept of 'social marketing' for health is now receiving increased interest in North America and Australia, where there have been successful programmes, for instance regarding stopping smoking. Whilst some advertising is necessary the main thrust of programmes relies on the wide availability of health products or services which the consumer wants and can afford, and the energetic use of public relations, and community action.

Appendix 4 contains an action guide to assist those health professionals who see a role for the media in their own health promotion activities, but who are unsure how to initiate or plan such a joint project. The various stages involved in the planning process are outlined. The guide assumes that an informed and realistic decision to approach the media has already been made. For example, there may be a need to communicate with a particular target group or to convey particular kinds of information. Obviously not every stage given is relevant for every project, nor is the order of 'events' sacrosanct, but the guide offers an agenda of questions that are worth considering.

Nutrition has been chosen as the example in the guide to illustrate how the model works in practice. This health education project is designed to alert people to the links between their own diet and their present and future health. It is based on an actual project currently in development, involving television, print, viewing groups and local radio. It should be stressed that such projects are ambitious, occasional and expensive – but they represent a growing area of activity for both broadcasters, and voluntary and professional organisations.

Recommendations

1. Initiatives using the mass media should wherever possible be planned jointly with health educators. The best results come when there are supportive programmes within the community and primary health care. Health agencies working with the media have a special responsibility to consult at local level to ensure maximum co-operation.

2. One year in the 1980s should be designated the 'Year of the Heart'. This could be in 1985 – the earliest feasible year, or a later year to

allow time for royal patronage, the special issue of postage stamps etc, to be arranged.

3. Campaigns for the prevention of coronary heart disease should include:

   (i) Regular press conferences at which senior doctors and scientists make major statements about heart disease prevention;

   (ii) Sponsorship of events mounted specifically with the purpose of publicising heart disease prevention.

4. An appropriate national body should give its seal of approval to cookery books, restaurants, hotels, hospitals, schools and establishments whose food is healthy; a 'greasy spoon' likewise could be awarded to others.

5. All over the world, bad news gets more coverage than good news. News coverage should therefore be encouraged of institutions, firms and individuals whose policies are damaging the cause of heart disease prevention.

6. The Coronary Prevention Group and others should lobby media organisations to appoint health correspondents and editors, nationally, regionally and locally. As part of this campaign, selected people in the media not yet so designated should be treated as such.

7. The Coronary Prevention Group or other appropriate national bodies should regularly publish a national newsletter. This should include a standard set of briefing documents, as well as special features. All material should be fully referenced.

8. The Health Education Council should sponsor four new National Press Awards for 'Best Health Coverage', in the following categories: national press, local press, magazines, broadcasting.

9. A Health Handbook should be published annually along the lines of the BBC Handbook. This should find a commercial publisher, and might be sponsored by the Health Education Council. Contents should include a directory of every type of health care resource and also chapters specifically relevant to that year.

10. The Health Education Council should commission an expanded version of the 'Handy Hints for Health Promoters' presented in Table II. This should be compiled by a small group of media professionals.

11. Directories should be compiled of all relevant and sympathetic media professionals and appropriate health scientists, promoters

and agencies. The Health Education Council should consider how it can improve communication between media and health professionals.

12. Each Regional Health Authority Press and Public Relations Department should identify one of its staff as having a special responsibility for health promotion and the prevention of coronary heart disease. Additional appointments may therefore be necessary.

13. Health promotion should be a standing item on the agenda of the meetings of the Regional Public Relations Officers, as a way of raising standards and encouraging development.

14. The BBC and IBA should be encouraged to produce by 1985 internal policy documents on 'Television and Safeguarding the Nation's Health', to cover all types of programmes, notably drama. This document should be compiled in the same way as the recent BBC report on television violence, with outside expert advice.

15. The effect of television on health should be the subject of a formal discussion or workshop within the normal structure of the 1984 Edinburgh Television Festival. A suggested title is 'How many Viewers did you Kill Today?'.

58

REFERENCES AND SUGGESTED FURTHER READING

Action on Smoking and Health (ASH) Health Education Council (1981). Smoking Prevention: *A Health Promotion Guide for the NHS.* London: ASH

Beattie A. (1983) *Health Education for the Prevention of Coronary Heart Disease.* Institute of Education, London University (unpublished)

Brent Health Authority (1982). *Food and Health Policy for Brent.* London: Brent HA

Health Education Council (1983). *Programmes for 1983–4.* London: Health Education Council

National Advisory Committee on Nutrition Education (1983). *Proposals for Nutritional Guidelines for Health Education in Britain.* London: Health Education Council

Physical Education Association of Great Britain and Northern Ireland (1979). *Guidelines for the Physical Education Curriculum.* London: PEA

Royal College of General Practitioners (1983). *Promoting Prevention.* Occasional Paper 22

Royal College of Physicians, British Cardiac Society (1976). Prevention of Coronary Heart Disease. *Journal of the Royal College of Physicians; 10:* 213ff

Royal College of Physicians (1983). *Health or Smoking?* London: Pitman

US Department of Health Education and Welfare (1979). *Healthy People.* The Surgeon General's Report on Health Promotion and Disease Prevention

US Department of Health and Human Services (1980). *Promoting Health Preventing Disease: Objectives for the Nation*

Wessex Positive Health Team (1983). *Exercise and Health: What Should the NHS be Doing?* Lifeline Report No 7. Winchester: Wessex Regional Health Authority

World Health Organization (1982). *Prevention of Coronary Heart Disease.* Report of a WHO Expert Committee. Technical Report Series 678. Geneva: WHO

Appendix 1
WORLD HEALTH ORGANIZATION
RECOMMENDATIONS
Summary of the recommendations of the WHO Expert Committee Report on the Prevention of Coronary Heart Disease. Technical Report Series No 678. Geneva: WHO 1982

1. In high incidence countries the majority of people have levels of major risk factors which are too high. Most cases of CHD occur among the large numbers who have moderate elevation of risk factors, not among the small number with high values. Only a mass (population) approach can help this larger group.

2. The relationships between habitual diet, blood cholesterol, lipoprotein levels and CHD are well established and are judged to be causal. In high-incidence countries a lowering of the population distribution of blood cholesterol is recommended through progressive changes in eating patterns. As a guideline, a population average value of under 200mg/dl (5.2mmol/dl) is likely to be associated with no more than a moderate frequency of CHD. Nutrient intakes for populations to achieve such levels involve limiting saturated fats to less than 10 per cent of calories, dietary cholesterol under 300mg/day average, and the avoidance of obesity. These are consistent with attractive and widely found eating patterns. Some of the reduction in saturated fat may be made up by mono- and poly-unsaturated fats. Present evidence on effectiveness and safety does not justify general advice to increase the intake of any particular fatty acids.

3. Even a small reduction in *average* blood pressure of the population could bring an important reduction in CHD. Based on the evidence as a whole it is recommended that populations should be encouraged to reduce consumption of salt in the direction of 5g daily or less. The importance of controlling obesity and excess alcohol consumption in the population is stressed.

4. Smoking, especially of cigarettes, contributes importantly to the occurrence of CHD. The first objective is that non-smoking should come to be regarded as normal behaviour, and strategies for achieving this are available. As far as CHD is concerned, present evidence does not support promotion of the so-called 'safer cigarette'.

5. Lack of physical activity relates to increased population levels of the major CHD risk factors, primarily through the high prevalence

of obesity. Population levels of obesity are importantly influenced by average energy expenditure. Regular exercise may help to reduce high blood pressure and blood cholesterol. A higher priority is therefore given to physical activity in CHD prevention than is justifiable simply by its association with CHD. Regular physical activity should be a part of usual daily life.

6. The underlying atherosclerotic process leading to mass CHD begins in youth, along with the appearance of its major risk characteristics, elevated blood pressure and cholesterol, and their associated risky behaviours, including smoking. Preventive measures need to start in childhood, so as to prevent development of these CHD precursors.

    National programme planning should be initiated for youth, as part of a comprehensive disease prevention and health promotion effort. Effective education programmes, including the prevention of smoking, are now available and should be adapted for local needs, implemented and then evaluated. Educated youth act as agents for improved health behaviour in the community.

Appendix 2
EXAMPLE OF A REGIONAL PLAN FOR THE PREVENTION OF CORONARY HEART DISEASE
(This has been prepared for a hypothetical average Region with 3 million population and 12 District Health Authorities)

Coronary heart disease is the major cause of premature death in the region today for both men and women. In 1981 the mortality rate for men aged 45–64 was 498 per 100,000 and for women it was 128 per 100,000. The situation is particularly alarming not only because of the cost in human terms and the considerable drain on scarce NHS resources but also because at least 25 per cent of the mortality and morbidity is thought to be preventable by the application of current knowledge regarding smoking, diet, exercise and hypertension. Numerous expert committees, nationally and internationally, have concluded that there is considerable scope for improvement and the dramatic decline in mortality in some other countries, notably the United States, Australia and Finland shows that progress is possible. Tables III and IV describe the scale of the problem in the region and the impact it has on health service resources.

The Regional Health Authority together with the Department of Health has concluded that the region should mount a major initiative over the next five years in heart disease prevention and that this activity should be the highest priority for NHS resources along with whatever each individual region decides.

The role of the Authority will be to:

(i) Define the priorities, strategy and mechanisms for the prevention of coronary heart disease

(ii) Ensure that District policies and programmes are established

(iii) Ensure that adequate resources are made available

(iv) Monitor the implementation of heart disease prevention programmes and progress towards the achievement of the Region's goal and specific objectives

(v) Provide operational support which Districts alone will not be able to provide: e.g. training, information, publicity and public relations

(vi) Encourage central government and national bodies (e.g. Health Education Council) to give the fullest support.

This Regional Plan seeks to set objectives for heart disease prevention programmes which concern not only reductions in mortality but also

TABLE III. Coronary Heart Disease Statistics (ICD 410–414) 1980 (calculated for an average region in England and Wales with a 3 million population)

		Age (years)		
MALE	All	25–44	45–64	65–74
1. Deaths*	5536	111	1585	1947
2. Deaths/100,000*	378	28	482	1583
3. Per cent deaths of all deaths*	31.1	21.4	39.5	33.7
4. General/acute hospital departures†	5148	435	2567	1347
5. General/acute hospital departures/10,000†	35.2	11	78	110
6. Average daily bed occupation†	178	10.7	63.8	44.6
7. Per cent of beds occupied of all admissions into general/acute beds†	4.6	2.9	8.1	5.0
8. Hospital costs per year, £1000s☆	£5,231	£314	£1,875	£1,311
FEMALE				
1. Deaths*	3945	18	433	1049
2. Deaths/100,000*	256	4.6	126	660
3. Per cent of all deaths*	22.3	5.2	18.4	26.8
4. General/acute hospital departures†	2541	128	682	751
5. General/acute hospital departures/10,000†	16.5	3.3	19.8	47.3
6. Average daily bed occupation†	161.5	2.0	18.5	34.0
7. Per cent of beds occupied of all admissions into general/acute beds†	2.5	0.4	2.2	2.8
8. Hospital costs per year, £1000s☆	£4,746	£59	£544	£999

* Source: OPCS

† Source: General Hospital Activity Analysis

☆ Column 6 x average cost per day of an acute bed in a non-teaching hospital with more than 100 beds (£80.51 at 1982/83 prices)

TABLE IV. Arterial Disease Statistics (ICD 401–405, 410–414, 430–438, 440) 1980 (calculated for an average region in England and Wales with a 3 million population)

		MALE All	25–44	Age (years) 45–64	65–74
1.	Deaths*	7459	139	1873	2566
2.	Deaths/100,000*	510	35	569	2095
3.	Per cent deaths of all deaths*	41.9	25.5	46.7	44.7
4.	General/acute hospital departures†	8687	610	3549	2600
5.	General/acute hospital departures/10,000†	59.4	15.4	107.8	212.3
6.	Average daily bed occupation†	524.9	16.9	115.9	167.16
7.	Per cent of beds occupied of all admissions into general/acute beds†	13.6	4.6	14.7	18.7
8.	Hospital costs per year, £1000s☆	£15,425	£497	£3,406	£4,912

FEMALE

		All	25–44	45–64	65–74
1.	Deaths*	7131	35	654	1651
2.	Deaths/100,000*	463	9	190	1040
3.	Per cent deaths of all deaths*	40.4	10.2	27.8	42.2
4.	General/acute hospital departures†	6608	299	1288	1799
5.	General/acute hospital departures/10,000†	42.9	7.7	37.4	113.3
6.	Average daily bed occupation†	1062.6	6.8	62.8	235.8
7.	Per cent of beds occupied of all admissions into general/acute beds†	16.6	1.3	7.4	19.4
8.	Hospital costs per year, £1000s☆	£31,226	£200	£1,845	£6,929

* Source: OPCS
† Source: General Hospital Activity Analysis
☆ Column 6 x average cost per day of an acute bed in a non-teaching hospital with more than 100 beds (£80.51 at 1982/83 prices)

changes in lifestyle which are known to be closely related to the occurrence of heart disease. It also states the activities which the Regional Health Authority will be undertaking to meet these objectives together with programmes that should be carried out by District Health Authorities. The final section describes the resources that will be made available to undertake this work.

The Region's Goal

The authority seeks to achieve similar reductions in premature deaths as experienced in some other developed countries, i.e. to seek to reduce deaths from coronary heart disease by at least 25 per cent amongst people aged 45 to 64 over the period 1984–1993 to fewer than 220 per 100,000 (ICD codes 410–414).

If achieved, this would result in a saving of about 500 deaths per year in the age group 45 to 64 in the Region. Reductions in deaths in other age groups would also be expected, together with falls in the levels of disability and handicap from arterial disease. In addition it would be expected that there would be savings in health service expenditure, lost output to Industry and National Insurance payments. In 1980 in the region the total drug bill for coronary heart disease was estimated at costing £12 million per year (25 per cent of the total drug bill), hospital admissions at least £10 million per year and lost output to Industry and National Insurance payments £33 million per year. Taking all forms of arterial disease including stroke, the costs are considerably greater, for example, hospital admissions amounted to £47 million per year (Table IV). Circulatory diseases are also the commonest reason for consultation in general practice, second only to respiratory disease. Consultation rates have been increasing over the last 10 years and in 1980 reached 800 per 1000 total population per year.

Because action directed at smoking, unhealthy nutrition, physical inactivity and hypertension will also contribute to the prevention of other major causes of ill health in the region, there should be considerable health and economic benefits in addition to those indicated above. The conditions concerned include stroke, cancer, respiratory disease, dental disease, mental and physical handicap and perinatal mortality.

Objectives

In order to achieve progress, the Authority believes that the pursuit of specific objectives is the key to success. These should concern the known risk factors for coronary heart disease at which intervention will be directed. The following objectives should be sought:

Smoking Prevention

(i) To encourage, motivate and help all those that do not smoke not to start, and all those who smoke to give up.

(ii) To assess the smoking status of all those aged 20–64 at least every five years so that specific support and help with cessation can be offered.

(iii) To promote non-smoking as the normal way of behaving, particularly in NHS premises and amongst NHS staff.

Healthy Nutrition

(i) To encourage the avoidance of obesity.

(ii) To promote a diet lower in fat, especially saturated fat, refined sugars and salt but which is high in fibre.

(iii) To accept the particular responsibility of the NHS in this field to its workforce and patients.

(iv) To assess the level of obesity (Body Mass Index greater than 29) in all those aged 20–64 at least every five years so that specific support and help with weight reduction can be offered.

Exercise Promotion

(i) To encourage the taking of sensible regular exercise as a part of the normal way of life.

(ii) To seek to increase the levels of physical activity in the community so that those aged under 64 undertake at least three periods of exercise per week which are brisk (i.e. aerobic) and sustained (i.e. 20 minutes or more).

(iii) To accept the particular NHS responsibility to its workforce in this field.

Hypertension Control

(i) To measure the blood pressure of all those aged 20–64 years at least every five years.

(ii) To offer advice on risk factor modification for those with hypertension.

(iii) To provide sustained and determined treatment for those with severe hypertension.

(iv) To ensure that the general public are aware of the importance of hypertension as a major risk factor for arterial disease which is capable of modification.

Targets

In developing programmes directed at these objectives, Districts will want to set target levels of achievement for given time periods. There will also be a need to set up an information base so that progress can be monitored. Clearly, targets have to be set, taking into account the current situation, the effectiveness of methods and resource assumptions.

The Authority would like District Health Authorities to comment and make other suggestions if appropriate on the following set of targets. These have been based on experience in other parts of this country and in other countries where considerable progress has occurred in modifying risk factors, e.g. Australia, Canada, Finland, USA. Given the commitment of health authorities and health professionals and moderate level of resources, the Authority believes that the following targets are achievable in the next 10 years. The Authority would also like suggestions on the timetabling for monitoring progress, namely, whether a five-year cycle is reasonable.

Smoking Prevention

For the period 1985—1995:

(i) To reduce the proportion of those aged 15—64 who smoke cigarettes by at least 1.5 per cent per annum on average (in 1982 38 per cent of adult men and 33 per cent of adult women smoked cigarettes).

(ii) To increase the proportion of those aged 15—64, who understand that smoking is one of the major risk factors for coronary heart disease and cancer by at least five per cent per annum on average (in 1981 the percentage was 36 per cent).

(iii) To increase the proportion of smokers aged 20—64, who have been offered smoking cessation counselling during the last three years by a primary care team member (e.g. general practitioner or health visitor) by at least five per cent per annum on average (baseline data not available — estimate 10 per cent).

(iv) To increase the proportion of those aged 15—64 who consider that smoking in public places, particularly where there are children, is anti-social by at least five per cent per annum on average (baseline data not available — estimate 10 per cent).

(v) To increase the proportion of 15–64 year olds who understand that parental smoking increases the risk of respiratory illness and smoking in their children by at least five per cent per annum on average (baseline data not available – estimate 20 per cent).

Healthy Nutrition

For the period 1985–1995:

(i) To reduce the proportion of those aged 15–64 with excess body weight (Body Mass Index greater than 25) by at least one per cent per annum on average (in 1981 the percentage was 36 per cent).

(ii) To reduce the mean total energy intake (including alcohol) from dietary fat of those aged 15–74 by at least 0.5 per cent per annum on average (in 1982 the percentage was 38 per cent).

(iii) To reduce the proportion of those aged 15–64 who routinely add salt to their food after cooking by at least two per cent per annum on average (baseline data not available – estimate 50 per cent).

(iv) To increase the proportion of those aged 15–64 who understand that obesity and diets which are high in fat, sugar and salt are hazardous to health, particularly coronary heart disease, by at least five per cent per annum on average (in 1981 the percentage was 36 per cent for obesity and nine per cent for diet).

(v) To increase the proportion of those seriously obese (Body Mass Index greater than 29) aged 20–64 who have been offered weight reduction counselling during the last three years by a primary care team member (e.g. general practitioner or health visitor) by at least five per cent per annum (baseline data not available – estimate 10 per cent).

Exercise Promotion

For the period 1985–1995:

(i) To increase the proportion of those aged 15–64 years who undertake brisk (aerobic) and sustained (over 20 minutes) exercise at least once per week by at least four per cent per annum on average (baseline data not available – estimate 30 per cent).

(ii) To increase the proportion of those aged 15–64 years who undertake brisk (aerobic) and sustained (over 20 minutes) exercise at least three times per week by at least two per cent per annum on average (baseline data not available – estimate 15 per cent).

(iii) To increase the proportion of those aged 15—64 years who understand what forms of exercise are beneficial to health, particularly
cardio-respiratory fitness, by at least five per cent per annum on
average (baseline data not available — estimate 20 per cent).

Hypertension Control

For the period 1985—1995:

(i) To increase the proportion of those aged 20—64 who have had
their blood pressure measured in the last five years by at least two
per cent per annum on average (baseline data not available —
estimate 50 per cent).

(ii) To increase the proportion of those aged 20—64 who are able to
state whether their blood pressure is in the normal range, or intermediate range (requiring regular monitoring and lifestyle modification), or high range (requiring treatment, regular monitoring and
lifestyle modification) by at least two per cent per annum on
average (baseline data not available — estimate 25 per cent).

(iii) To increase the proportion of those aged 15—64 who understand
raised blood pressure is a major risk factor for arterial disease by
at least five per cent per annum on average (in 1981 the percentage
was five per cent).

(iv) To increase the proportion of those aged 15—64 who understand
that stress reduction, avoidance of obesity, regular exercise and
moderate salt and fat intake may lessen the risk of hypertension
by at least five per cent per annum on average (baseline data not
available — estimate five per cent).

(v) To increase the proportion of those aged 15—64 who understand
that raised blood pressure does not normally produce symptoms
and that blood pressure should be measured at least every five
years, by at least five per cent per annum on average (baseline
data not available — estimate five per cent).

Monitoring

A key feature of this strategy will be careful monitoring to see whether
the agreed targets have been achieved. Therefore a new information
base will need to be established based on periodic community surveys.
Simple, reliable low cost survey techniques are currently being developed
for the type of self reported information, required for the monitoring
of the targets proposed above. In order to assure comparability between

Districts and over time, the Authority considers that it has an important role in the collection of the information in close collaboration with District Health Authorities. Comparability with other regions will be sought.

Implementing Regional Programmes

A small inter-disciplinary advisory group will be established comprising regional and district officers, health care professionals, and the Health Education Council staff responsible for mass media initiatives in the region. This will be a subgroup of the Regional Health Promotion Team. Duties will consist of:

- giving expert advice on heart disease prevention programmes
- co-ordinating the District activities with the Health Education Council, DHSS, Sports Council, radio, television and newspapers;
- establishing a data base for monitoring progress in achieving the stated objectives;
- providing operational support for Districts;
- organising training courses for authority chairs and members, chief officers and health professionals in consultation with Districts.

To help undertake this work, it is hoped that a new appointment of a Regional Health Promotion Officer with special responsibilities for heart disease prevention will be made jointly between the Health Education Council and the Regional Health Authority. The duties will be to service the advisory group and be one of the channels through which its duties are carried out. As a consequence of the joint appointment, it is hoped that the officer will be responsible for planning and implementing the Council's funded mass media campaigns.

The regional officer will receive secretarial services from the Authority and will be supported closely by the Regional Press and Public Relations Department. It is anticipated that the Health Education Council will allocate £300,000 per annum to mass media campaigns in the region (i.e. 10 pence per head of total population per year).

The Authority's Statistics and Information Division will undertake periodic measurements of knowledge, attitude, behaviour and health status in the community relevant to the risk factors for coronary heart disease. This new resource will be partly met by a re-allocation of existing staff time within the Division and partly by the appointment of additional staff. In addition the Authority will investigate the possibility of using private sector organisations who specialise in community surveys (e.g. market research and public opinion poll companies).

The Authority's Training Division, in close collaboration with the Regional Advisory Group, will organise training courses on heart disease prevention. Programmes will be published annually.

In the same way that the Authority's activities on heart disease prevention will be scrutinised in the annual ministerial review, attention will also be paid to it in the regular meetings of Regional and District chairs and officers.

At national level, the chairs and chief officers will press for ways in which the socio-economic environment could be improved to promote healthy lifestyles such as restricting cigarette advertising, implementing food labelling and developing a national nutrition policy.

District Activities

District Health Authorities will be expected to produce an annual plan for the prevention of coronary heart disease. This should:

- define the policies and programmes in accord with the Regional Strategy. These should be stated in terms of the four key risk factors (smoking, hypertension, unhealthy nutrition and physical inactivity);

- describe the infrastructure which will be developed to implement the programmes;

- describe the resources (manpower etc) that will be made available;

- indicate the support required from Regional Health Authority, Health Education Council and other bodies;

- define the timing of the programmes;

- provide a statement of the progress made.

The formation of an inter-disciplinary heart disease prevention team at District level is strongly recommended. Each Team might include a community physician, senior administrator, senior nursing officer, district health education officer, consultant physician, general practitioner, local authority representative (e.g. recreation manager), education authority representative (e.g. senior education adviser). The Team's task will be to plan programmes in line with Regional objectives and to manage a specially allocated budget to promote healthy lifestyles and risk avoidance. This fund would be provided by the RHA as a pump-priming grant for five years and could be used to develop activities at primary care level and in the community such as with schools, youth services, voluntary agencies, employers, etc.

There are two integrated approaches which are seen to be the cornerstones of action to prevent coronary heart disease. The first concerns the extension of primary care into the control of obesity and hypertension, and into smoking cessation. The second requires a community approach on a total population basis. The District Team alone can only provide a steering or co-ordinating role and cannot hope to have the sensitivity for local needs that more informal and locally based teams will have. Neighbourhood health strategies are crucial to the WHO's goal of Health for All by the Year 2,000 as they are more likely to provide a more sensitive framework for local planning, commitment and action. Neighbourhood health promotion groups for heart disease prevention are therefore recommended using health or community centres as a focal point for joint professional and community interaction.

There will be a need therefore for a Health Education/Promotion Officer (Community Development) and a Primary Care Team Liaison Person to develop initiatives at District level. These may require special appointments. The former will be responsible for stimulating and winning the support of the community, industry and local authorities. Their wishes and views could be incorporated into programmes (e.g. regarding the provision of nutritionally sound meals in schools and workplaces, the expansion of exercise facilities, promoting non-smoking in public places, establishment of self-help groups for slimming and stop-smoking). The latter appointment, who could be a sessional general practitioner, will be responsible for encouraging and advising general practitioners, health visitors and community nurses in activities appropriate for Primary Care Teams.

It is expected that an expansion of the activities of the District Health Education Service will be required. Any development would be for local consideration, taking into account the activities of the Health Education Council at regional level.

Districts will be expected to develop their Occupational Health Services facilities to ensure that NHS employees lead the District's population in the achievement of the agreed targets.

This reflects:

- the relative ease of implementing health promotion programmes for a defined population working within the NHS;

- the important exemplar role of NHS staff in the community and their potential as health educators.

Organisational changes within NHS premises will be necessary to support NHS workplace-based programmes, e.g. provision of no-smoking areas, exercise facilities and changing rooms, and healthy nutrition.

Resource Allocation

In view of the priority attached to heart disease prevention, the Authority together with the Department of Health have made a special allocation for the development of programmes. This pump-priming fund amounts to £630,000 per annum for a five year period. This will be allocated as follows:

(i) £30,000 per annum will be used for the appointment of the Regional Officer and statistical/monitoring support at Regional level.

(ii) Twenty pence per head of total population per annum for five years will be available to Districts to support heart disease prevention initiatives. Funding will be released by the Authority on the production of costed programmes. Districts will also be expected to make existing resources available for initiatives. It is for this reason that the Authority will be seeking at least a 'pound for pound' match from within current District allocations.

Appendix 3
EXAMPLE OF A DISTRICT PLAN FOR THE
PREVENTION OF CORONARY HEART DISEASE
(This has been prepared for a hypothetical average District of
250,000 population)

This plan has been developed after full and lengthy discussion with all those health professionals concerned with the prevention of coronary heart disease, and has been endorsed by the District Health Authority and its advisory committees, the Local Medical Committee and the Community Health Council.

This District supports the initiative mounted by DHSS and the RHA for a concerted attack on coronary heart disease prevention and agrees this should receive the highest priority along with whatever each individual district decides. It has therefore adopted the objectives and suggested targets contained in the Regional Plan.

In developing heart disease prevention programmes, two strategies will be advanced. One concerns the extension of Primary Care Team activities. The other concerns the development of community approaches towards modifying risk behaviour based on the experience of the Stanford and North Karelia programmes. This will involve close collaboration with non-NHS bodies such as local authorities, industry and commerce, voluntary organisations, etc.

District programmes have been developed for four key risk factors:

- smoking
- unhealthy nutrition
- physical inactivity
- hypertension

The school age population, young people, parents with young families and those in employment have been identified as target groups.

The District comprises several geographically identifiable communities which are distinct and diverse in a number of ways. It is accepted, therefore, that to be effective programmes need to be developed by and implemented through these communities. Informal neighbourhood teams will need to be set up comprising both professional and lay membership as they are more likely to provide a more sensitive framework for local planning, commitment and action. Nevertheless there is a need for a steering and co-ordinating group at District level which will ensure progress both managerially and politically.

1. District Heart Disease Prevention Team

An interdisciplinary heart disease prevention Team will therefore be set up comprising:

District Medical Officer
District Administrator
District Health Education Officer
Director of Nursing Services – or senior nurse (Community Unit)
Consultant Physician
General Practitioner (also the part time Primary Care Team Liaison Person)
Health Education Officer (Community Development)
Senior Officer of the Recreation Department of the Local Authority
Senior Officer of the Education Department of the Local Authority
Trades Union representative
Voluntary organisation representative
DHA Member (who is also a member of the Local Authority, and who will chair the Team)

The Terms of Reference will be:

(i)   To advise the Health Authority on heart disease prevention;

(ii)   To promote and implement programmes of heart disease prevention through individuals of the group;

(iii)   To stimulate the formation of neighbourhood teams for 'healthy living' based on health or community centres incorporating professional and lay membership;

(iv)   To initiate environmental and organisational change to support heart disease prevention programmes;

(v)   To provide in-service training and stimulus for health professionals and others concerned with heart disease prevention;

(vi)   To assess the effectiveness of those programmes implemented;

(vii)   To monitor the programmes with particular reference to the agreed targets in conjunction with the Regional Health Authority;

(viii) To receive applications from groups within and outside the NHS for grants from a specially formed fund.

2. Resources for Heart Disease Prevention

The RHA has offered the sum of 20 pence per head of total population per annum for the development of programmes in the District, as a pump-priming initiative for five years. This is on the basis that the

Authority matches the amount from within its own resources. The District has agreed to claim the sum available by obtaining some additional resources from some non-recurring money it has available from a delayed capital programme and realignment of some staff in the community health services (i.e. health visitors, medical officers and clerical officers). In addition to the appointment of a Health Education/Promotion Officer (Community Development) and a Primary Care Team Liaison Person, the Authority has set up a special fund to provide grants to any organisation/group wishing to undertake heart disease prevention work. This amounts to £30,000 for the first year. Applications are therefore invited for grants between £100 and £5,000 and should be sent to the secretary of the District Heart Disease Prevention Fund.

Grants might be given for:

Providing 'top-ups' to enable larger group practices to employ a 'prevention practice nurse';

Supporting the work of stop-smoking and slimming self-help groups;

Improving resources in the District Health Education Unit;

Sponsoring community exercise events;

Providing incentives for projects at school and in the workplace;

Holding training days for NHS staff;

Organising high profile public meetings;

Providing speakers for community clubs, works organisations, etc;

Stimulating and developing appropriate Further Education Courses held under the auspices of the Education Authority;

Helping general practices to produce annual reports of the health profiles of their populations.

3. Primary Care Team Activities

General practitioners, health visitors and community nurses will be visited by the Primary Care Team Liaison Person who will seek the active support of members of Primary Care Teams. The feasibility of realigning some of the work of health visitors will be discussed. The possibility of group practices employing an additional nurse who will be suitably trained in heart disease prevention work will also be considered. Seventy per cent of this nurse's salary normally would be paid by the Family Practitioner Committee under the existing arrangements for ancillary staff.

It may be possible for the remaining 30 per cent (less income tax)

payable to be provided from the District Heart Disease Prevention Fund.
Programmes at primary care level might consist of routinely calling up
patients aged 20–64 every five years for blood pressure, height and
weight measurement, and counselling on lifestyle factors such as
smoking, exercise and nutrition. A simple risk factor screening questionnaire might be used (e.g. Canadian Evalulife questionnaire). Regular
smoking cessation and slimming self-help groups would be held by the
practice nurse or health visitor. They would receive appropriate training
in group work.

The Liaison Person will not only play an important part in winning
the co-operation of primary care teams but will also have a continuing
role to play in their training, maintaining their interest and enthusiasm
and collecting information. Another important task will also be to keep
the Teams aware of all community-based programmes, perhaps through
the use of a newsletter.

The Community Health Services will also play their part in supporting
District programmes. Health education relevant to heart disease prevention will be undertaken wherever possible, e.g. during school medical
examinations, pre-school visits and developmental assessments, and in
family planning clinics.

4. Community Development

The Health Education/Promotion Officer (Community Development)
will be the spearhead of heart disease prevention activities within the
community. The initial task will be to win support of industry and
commerce, voluntary organisations, community health council members,
and community leaders (e.g. teachers, clergymen, politicians). It will
also be important to establish liaison with other workers who have a
role in implementing programmes. These include occupational health
staff (to undertake work-based activities), recreation managers (to
develop exercise facilities), environmental health officers (to promote
non-smoking as the norm), social workers (to help at-risk individuals
and families) and youth leaders (to reach young people not in contact
with Primary Care Teams).

The work will be reactive (i.e. opportunistic) as well as proactive and
will require imagination and entrepreneurial skills. The varying cultural
and socio-economic features within the District must be taken into
account in all plans. Activities will be aided by small grants from the
Heart Disease Prevention Fund but it is expected that modest fund
raising would also be undertaken (e.g. sponsored fun runs).

Together with the Primary Care Team Liaison Person, a key task will
be to stimulate the formation of neighbourhood teams for heart disease

prevention, comprising professional and lay membership. These it is hoped will be the focal point of community action at local level.

5. District Health Education Service

It is recognised that the District Health Education Service is already under considerable pressure given its present resources. The Authority would not want other educational programmes to suffer as a result of the District's initiative on heart disease prevention. Services directed at immunisation, ante-natal care, child health, accident prevention, dental health, fertility control and cancer screening still require important contributions from the Health Education Service. Nevertheless, as many of their current activities concern risk factors relevant to heart disease prevention, the Health Education Service will work closely with the Heart Disease Prevention Team. The District Health Education Officer will be a core member of the Team.

In addition to the contributions from the Community Development Officer, the District Health Education Service will support the programme as follows:

(i)   Develop and provide health education materials for Primary Care Teams and community groups. If additional resources are required, these will be found from the District Heart Disease Prevention Fund.

(ii)   Work with school and adult education teachers, particularly in the fields of smoking, nutrition and exercise (e.g. advising on the structure and content of courses, and the training of teachers).

(iii)   Undertake evaluation of programmes.

(iv)   Hold training courses for NHS staff and others.

(v)   Liaise closely with the Health Education Council on regional mass media campaigns.

(vi)   Initiate organisational changes within NHS, local authority and other premises which will support programmes, e.g. provision of non-smoking areas, exercise facilities and changing rooms, healthy nutrition in canteens, etc.

(vii)   Undertake other activities which will support the programmes.

6. Smoking Prevention Programmes

In addition to the regional mass media programmes of the Health Education Council, which will be developed in close collaboration with the

District, the following activities will be undertaken:

Primary Care Teams will be encouraged to:

(i)   identify opportunistically and preferably systematically every five years those adults aged 20–64 who smoke;

(ii)   offer one-to-one stop-smoking counselling and literature;

(iii)   mail health education material on smoking-cessation regularly to smokers;

(iv)   organise regular smoking cessation self-help groups (practice based);

(v)   refer highly dependent smokers wishing to give up smoking but who have not responded to practice based programmes to a special District smoking-cessation clinic run by a psychologist.

Community Development activities will consist of:

(i)   providing self-help leaflets and kits to those smokers who would like to give up;

(ii)   encouraging the development of smoking cessation self help groups;

(iii)   increasing no-smoking areas in hospitals;

(iv)   action to improve smoking restrictions in local authority and other premises;

(v)   surveying smoking in public places and subsequently publicising the need for improvements;

(vi)   assessing the extent to which cigarettes are sold to children under 16 years, and subsequently publicising the need for greater restrictions;

(vii)   promoting 'non-smoking as the norm' as opportunities arise.

7. Healthy Nutrition Programmes

In addition to mass media programmes of the Health Education Council, which will be developed in close collaboration with the District, the following activities will be undertaken:

Primary Care Teams will be encouraged to:

(i)   identify opportunistically or preferably systematically every five years those aged 20–64 who are obese (Body Mass Index greater than 29);

(ii)   offer one-to-one counselling and literature regarding weight reduction;

(iii)   organise regular slimming self help groups (practice based);

(iv)   refer obese patients wishing to lose weight but who have not responded to practice-based programmes to the District Dietetic Service.

Community Development activities will consist of:

(i)   providing self-help leaflets and kits on healthy nutrition;

(ii)   encouraging development of slimming self help groups;

(iii)   improving nutrition policies in hospitals;

(iv)   action to improve nutrition policies in local authority premises, schools, colleges, large work-places, etc;

(v)   promoting 'healthy nutrition' as opportunities arise.

8. Exercise Promotion Programmes

In addition to mass media programmes of the Health Education Council, which will be developed in close collaboration with the District, the following activities will be undertaken:

Primary Care Teams will be encouraged to:

(i)   offer counselling and literature, opportunistically, on the benefits of exercise and what suitable methods and facilities exist;

(ii)   set an example as 'role models' (e.g. organising practice-based keep-fit, jogging groups).

Community Development activities will consist of:

(i)   providing self-help leaflets and kits on sensible exercise;

(ii)   encouraging and sponsoring community based exercise events;

(iii)   encouraging improvements in work-based facilities and opportunities so that those at work can take exercise in free time (especially NHS and Local Authority staff);

(iv)   encouraging the expansion of community exercise facilities and opportunities (e.g. longer opening hours of recreation centres, use of school facilities and village halls, opening of nature trails, etc).

9. Hypertension Control Programmes

In addition to mass media programmes of the Health Education Council (i.e. concerning salt, fat, obesity) which will be developed in close collaboration with the District, the following activities will be undertaken.

Primary Care Teams will be encouraged to:

(i)   identify opportunistically or preferably systematically every five years those adults aged 20–64 with raised blood pressure;

(ii)   offer one-to-one counselling and literature to those with hypertension concerning modification of risk factors (e.g. exercise, salt, obesity, stress) and to monitor regularly;

(iii)   offer drug treatment to those with severe hypertension.

Community Development activities will consist of:

(i)   increasing knowledge in the community of the important risk factors for hypertension/coronary heart disease;

(ii)   increasing knowledge about the importance of early detection and treatment of hypertension, which is often without symptoms.

10. NHS Occupational Health Services

The NHS is a community and great emphasis is placed on the exemplar role of those working for the Health Service. There is need, therefore, for NHS staff to take a lead in adopting healthy lifestyles. Special programmes, along the lines presented above for the general population, will be developed by the Authority's Occupational Health Staff. These will be as complementary as possible to developments occurring elsewhere in the community.

Appendix 4
ACTION GUIDE – *SO YOU THINK YOU WANT TO USE THE MEDIA?*

> *This guide assumes that:*
> Nature of the problem has been identified
> Ideological, financial and ethical constraints have been recognised
> Aims and objectives have been agreed
> Content and method discussed
> Use of the media has been agreed as an appropriate method

THE MODEL	EXPLANATION	WORKED EXAMPLE ON FOOD AND HEALTH
1. What is your goal?	Be realistic – the media can inform and change attitudes (at least for a while) but don't expect to be able to change behaviour unless other factors are also working towards this end.	Project has three aims: • Encourage people to take into account up-to-date nutritional advice when deciding what food to buy. • Enable food 'caterers' (the role played by those who purchase and prepare food for themselves and others) to be aware of what influences their decision and constrains their choice. • Alert them to the opportunities to influence political and commercial policy making.
2. What strategy have you planned?	It should be a strategy that has elements of a campaign in it – reaching as large a number of people as possible and concentrating on raising awareness and altering attitudes. It usually involves a complex integration of different media.	Following publication of the NACNE report, encourage public debate and individual thought by co-ordinating transmission of specially commissioned TV series with print materials designed for both individual and group use, and various forms of local activity.

3. Why does this strategy assume the use of the mass media?

The use of transmitted media is usually justified on the grounds of the wide or targeted audience they can reach. Print may reach fewer people but those who do read it may pay more attention to it! Market Research data can be particularly useful here.

Because it is well known that food programmes and publications are popular with a large and broad sector of the British public (particularly women) and the mass media are therefore a cost-effective means of communicating with a substantial proportion of this target group.

4. What function do you see broadcasting fulfilling within the total project?

In particular, what can TV and radio do that is less well done in print or too expensive by other means? E.g. updating, stimulating discussion, raising awareness of values and attitudes held, identifying political and economic aspects of issues, enhancing audience identification with those involved in the situations by use of case studies and drama.

- Providing information on up-to-date nutritional knowledge and advice.
- Raising awareness of the values and attitudes that lie behind the selection of food purchases.
- Illustrating, by case studies, the role of government and industry in establishing food and agricultural policy.
- Suggesting strategies for making informed decisions on food when shopping and cooking.

5. What broadcast medium could best fulfil this function?

Take advice about 'horses for courses'. NB many people think of TV first and don't even consider other media; it might be better to consider TV last on the grounds of its high cost and ephemeral nature.

Either TV or radio could cover these issues, but TV likely to reach larger audience and achieve greater impact. Material also usable as video after transmission.

6. How would the broadcast elements be integrated with the other components of the project?

Because TV and radio are so ephemeral you should certainly consider print material – links with newspapers (national and local), magazines, response mailers and booklets, publishing a specially commissioned book. You need to pay particular attention to how individuals and groups will know about and use the various components if they wish to.

Series would be supported by free booklets, published book and programme notes for use by groups. Long term possibility of building videos into more structured learning package. Thought given to ways of alerting particular networks to availability of the materials and possibility of forming viewing/discussion groups.

7. Whose support, collaboration or partnership would you need to set up the project?	Field networks, like local health education officers, WI, National Housewives Register, Samaritans, Trades Unions, Community groups, charities, pressure groups, etc. And obviously broadcasters if your project requires radio or TV components, and broadcast support systems. Possibly distance learning institutions (e.g. Open University, National Extension College).	Health education professionals and organisations (e.g. HEC, College of Health) for expert advice, access to networks and possibly financial support. Consultants in technical and specialist areas, e.g. nutritionists, agricultural economists, etc. Broadcasters (Channel 4) and Broadcast Support Services. Open University Community Education Unit.
8. Where will you find the necessary resources? • people? • money?	Money *is* important but so is finding the people who have the necessary skills you need. Programme budgets normally come wholly or partly from broadcasting funds. Print material can often be sponsored but is sometimes commercially viable. Specialist organisations that do not have substantial funds will usually have access to experts either on staff or in a voluntary capacity.	People either employed for their expert skills, or brought in at no cost because the work constitutes part of their existing job description. Programme budgets either entirely from broadcast funds or co-production. Additional funds possibly raised from foundations or relevant organisations, e.g. for research.
9. What steps do you need to take to ensure a shared understanding of the goal — and to set objectives?	A 'new readers start here' update, or a workshop to establish shared assumptions, values or 'style'.	Planning meetings or seminars for all parties to exchange opinions and approaches, hear expert or specialist views, consider existing research data. Discussion papers prepared by various members of planning group.
10. How will you evaluate the effectiveness of the project?	The earlier you start to think about this, the easier it is to get advice. Where possible formative research can feed into the production process at an early stage (e.g. Pilots). Failing which, involving researchers in the development stage will help you and then set realistic objectives for this project as a whole.	Existing research considered (see above) and research consultants approached. Funding for research built into project budget if possible. Potential researchers involved in early planning stage.

11. How are tasks allocated between partners?

Does everyone know who is responsible for doing what — and when it will be done by?

Programme consultants for each programme identified; writers of print material agreed; contacts with networks established and liaison with transmission outlets maintained.

12. How do you formalise these agreements?
• financial
• contractual
• copyright
• editorial responsibility

Get it all in writing and ensure that all parties concerned see it. If appropriate, take legal advice.

Negotiations on legal and budgetary matters take place. All queries on rights resolved as early as possible. Each form of editorial involvement and final responsibility clarified.

13. How will the project be managed?
• operational objectives established?
• progress monitored?

Make sure everyone knows who is responsible for what — and by when. Build in routine progress checks.

Schedule agreed and circulated. Responsibility for individual tasks allocated. Regular meetings to report and review work in progress.

14. How will you mobilise the networks in the field?

This can take more effort than initially anticipated. Patience, legwork, and careful negotiation of the collaboration are needed. Responsibility for these negotiations will vary according to who in the planning group has the best contacts.

Advance information given in newsletters, etc. National or regional briefing sessions planned. Viewing groups set up if desirable.

15. How will you publicise the project to the target audience?

Rather than general publicity can you use existing networks to channel publicity to your target audience? Adequate advance information is crucial for any planned educational usage.

National and local press coverage. Publicity via broadcasters' press/PR system. Special events/ launch. On air trails.

16. How will you orchestrate the delivery?
    - synchronise transmission and publication deadlines?
    - co-ordinate back-up arrangements?
    - have ready relevant evaluation components?

    Transmission dates should be sacred, but rarely can be guaranteed. You may need to frighten printers with 'time is of the essence' contract — no money if it's not there by the deadline. Are you sure the phone lines will be adequately manned?

    Finalise publishing and transmission dates as early as possible, to enable maximum advance notice to the field. Anticipate audience response and organise back-up accordingly. Organise viewing groups where appropriate. Plan survey or interview strategy for research purposes.

17. How will you implement appropriate post-project evaluation?

    Don't leave it too late; much of the effect of the media is short term! Focus on measurable outcomes rather than general response whenever possible, and base these on the realistic objectives you set at the outset.

    Quantitative and qualitative data collected — partly from usual audience research, also from specially commissioned research. If possible, some assessment of broadcast support operation and longer term evaluation of print material. Attempt to compare short term 'immediate' response with longer term behavioural change, if any.

18. Identify scapegoats?

    The projects rarely fulfil all expectations; identify process related improvements that could be implemented in future projects.

    Assess how well the various parties co-operated and decide whether such arrangements have long-term potential. If things have gone wrong — why, and how could they have been avoided?

19. How will you disseminate your findings to improve the next phase and for other goal setters?

    Much of what you learn both from successes and mistakes should be of use to other people on other projects. Differentiate between the specific operational lessons learned on this project, that may or may not be transferable, and broader lessons learned about general practice for co-operative ventures of this sort. Publicise your conclusions where appropriate.

    Evaluation/research report completed and circulated to relevant groups/individuals. First-hand accounts of project published within each organisation for future reference.